THIS JOURNAL BELONGS TO:

_____

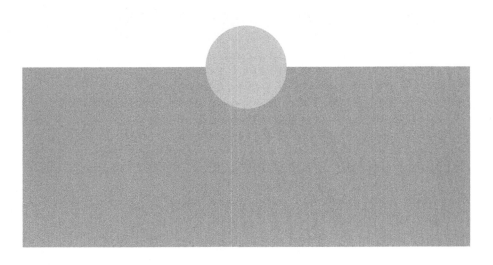

HOW TO USE
THIS JOURNAL

This journal was created by a Licensed Professional Counselor after seeing a very common need for her clients to practice improving their emotional awareness and connection to themselves.

Utilizing a variety of evidence-based techniques from Cognitive Behavioral Therapy(CBT), Dialectical Behavioral Therapy(DBT), mindfulness, Art Therapy, and concepts from Nonviolent Communication, this journal provides you with a daily practice to consciously and mindfully develop your connection to yourself.

- "I FEEL" - Tap into yourself and give name to the emotion(s) of the day. Use the emotion wheel provided at the beginning of this journal to help build your emotional vocabulary, or use your own word to identify.
- "ABOUT/BECAUSE" - Be specific in communicating the context and what has triggered or influenced the emotion.
- "I NEED" - Positive feelings come when our needs are being met, while uncomfortable feelings come when they aren't. Try to identify if there is anything you are needing by using the list of needs at the beginning of this journal, or identify your own.
- "I CHOOSE" - You can choose what actions you will or will not take in response to these emotions. Will you communicate your needs? Will you take a deep breath to relax? Will you choose to forgive? Will you take action to make sure your needs are met? You are in control of your actions and emotions.
- "ART" - Where in your body do you feel the emotion(s)? What physical sensation(s) does it give you? Do your fists clench? Does your heart beat faster? If you could see the emotion(s), what would it look like? What shape? What color? What texture? Use the provided space to draw and try to get to know the emotion(s) and allow yourself to truly feel and understand them without pushing them away.

date: 3/3/22

Today, I feel angry, disappointed, lonely

about my friends not inviting me to
hang out with them

because it makes me feel left out and
think they might not like me or care about me.

I need reassurance, friendship, acceptance
inclusion, consideration

I choose to take 3 deep breaths, calmly
communicate my feelings and needs, forgive

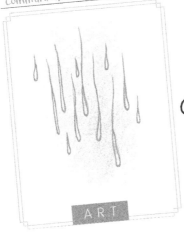

ART

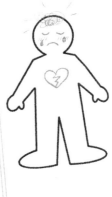

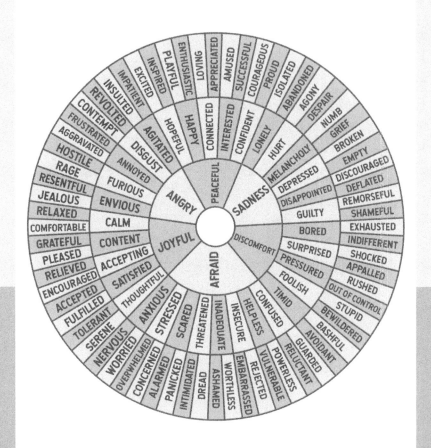

EMOTION WHEEL

LIST OF NEEDS

ACCEPTANCE
ACCOUNTABILITY
ACKNOWLEDGMENT
AFFECTION
APPRECIATION
AUTHENTICITY
AUTONOMY
BALANCE
CHOICE
CLARITY
COMFORT
COMMUNITY
COMPASSION
COMPETENCE
CONNECTION
CONSIDERATION
CONTRIBUTION
CREATIVITY
DEPENDABILITY
EASE
EMPATHY

EFFICIENCY
EQUALITY
FLEXIBILITY
FREEDOM
FRIENDSHIP
FUN
GROWTH
HARMONY
HEALTH
HELP
HONESTY
HOPE
INCLUSION
INSPIRATION
INTIMACY
KINDNESS
LOVE
MEANING
MOURNING
NURTURANCE
ORDER
PARTICIPATION
PEACE
PLAY
POWER
PREDICTABILITY
PRIVACY
PROTECTION
PURPOSE

REASSURANCE
RESPECT
RESPONSIBILITY
REST
RELAXATION
SAFETY
SECURITY
SELF-EXPRESSION
SHARED REALITY
SPACE
SPONTANEITY
STIMULATION
STRUCTURE
SUPPORT
TO BE HEARD
TO BE SEEN
TO MATTER & BELONG
TRUST
UNDERSTANDING
WELL-BEING

date:_____

Today, I feel_____

about _____

_____

because_____

_____

I need_____

_____

I choose_____

_____

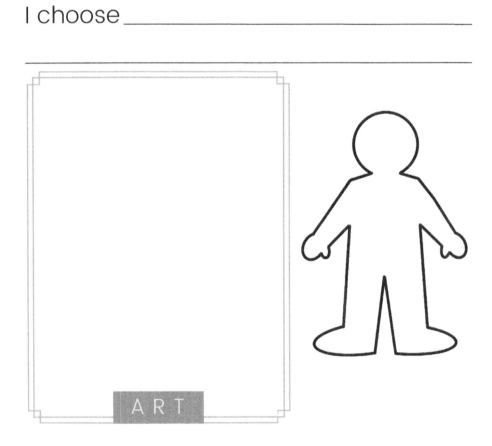

ART

date:_____

Today, I feel_____

about _____

_____

because_____

_____

I need_____

_____

I choose _____

_____

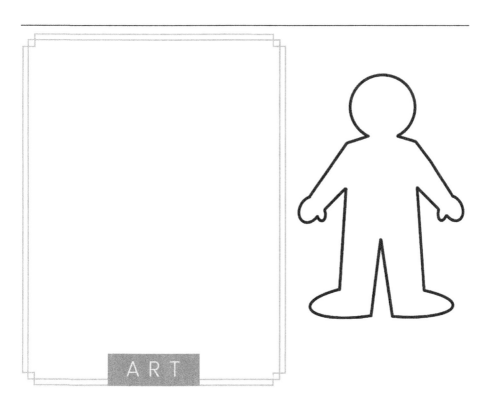

ART

date:_____

Today, I feel_____

about _____

_____

because_____

_____

I need_____

_____

I choose_____

_____

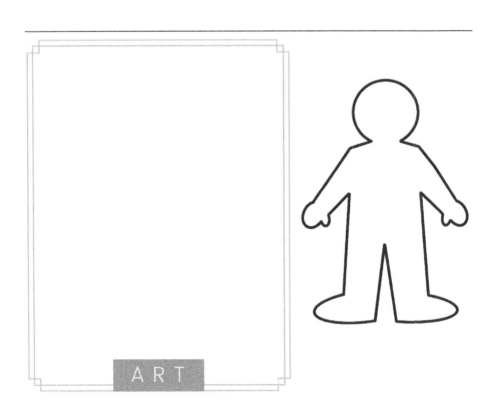

ART

date:_____

Today, I feel_____

about _____

_____

because_____

_____

I need_____

_____

I choose _____

_____

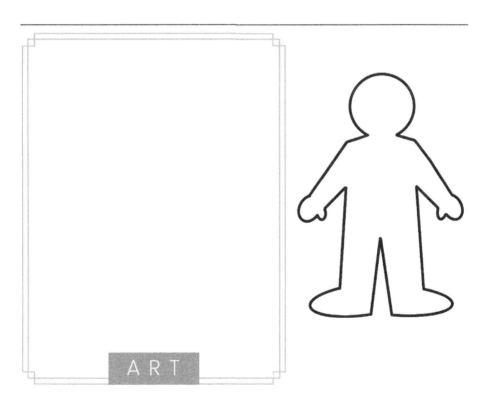

ART

date:_____

Today, I feel_____

about _____

_____

because_____

_____

I need_____

_____

I choose _____

_____

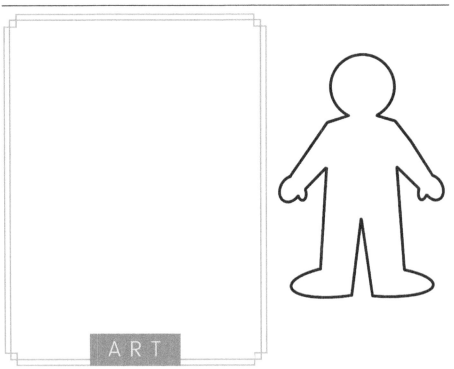

ART

date:_____

Today, I feel_____

about _____

_____

because_____

_____

I need_____

_____

I choose _____

_____

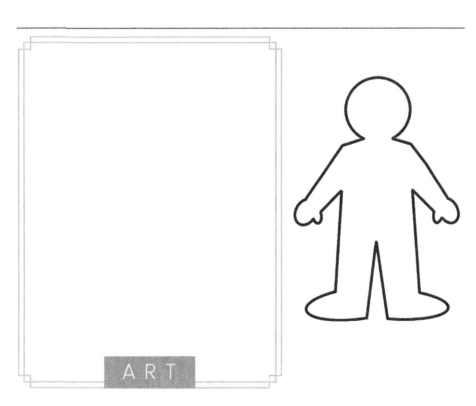

ART

date:_____

Today, I feel_____

about _____

_____

because_____

_____

I need_____

_____

I choose _____

_____

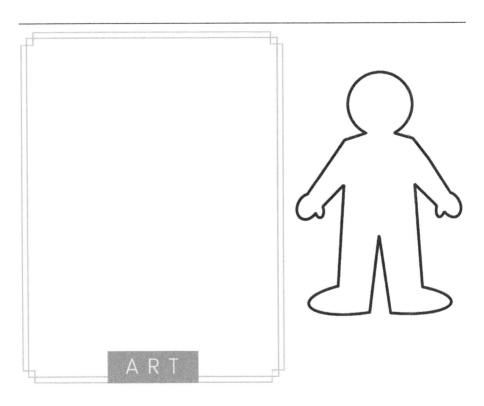

ART

date:_____

Today, I feel_____

about _____

_____

because_____

_____

I need_____

_____

I choose_____

_____

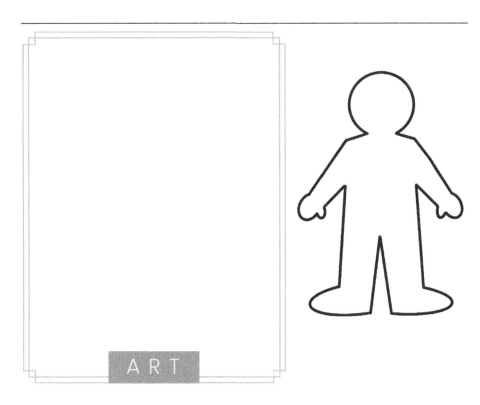

ART

date:_____

Today, I feel_____

about _____

_____

because_____

_____

I need_____

_____

I choose_____

_____

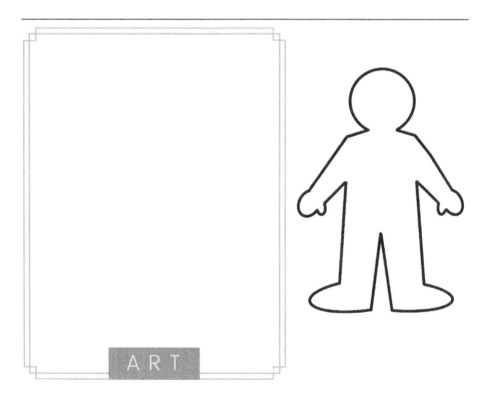

ART

date:_____

Today, I feel_____

about _____

_____

because_____

_____

I need_____

_____

I choose _____

_____

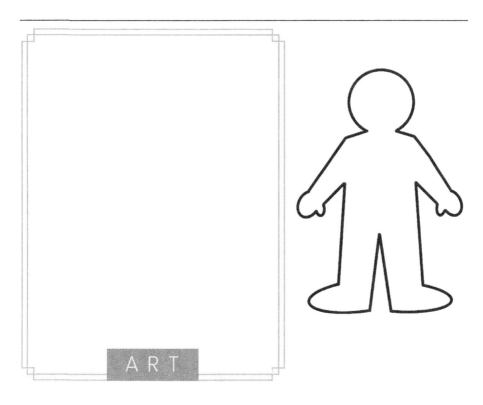

ART

date:_____

Today, I feel_____

about _____

_____

because_____

_____

I need_____

_____

I choose_____

_____

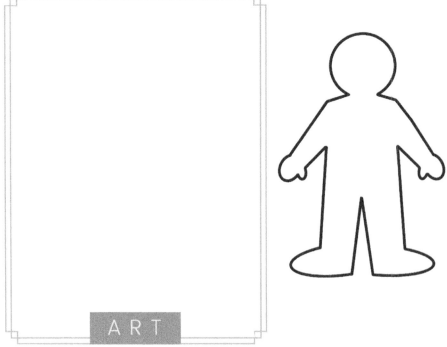

ART

date:_____

Today, I feel_____

about _____

_____

because_____

_____

I need_____

_____

I choose _____

_____

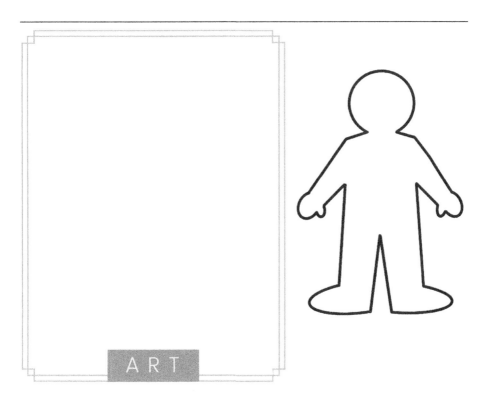

ART

date:_____

Today, I feel_____

about _____

_____

because_____

_____

I need_____

_____

I choose_____

_____

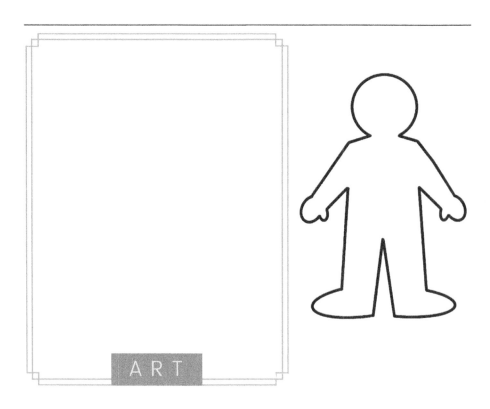

ART

date:_____

Today, I feel_____

about _____

_____

because_____

_____

I need_____

_____

I choose_____

_____

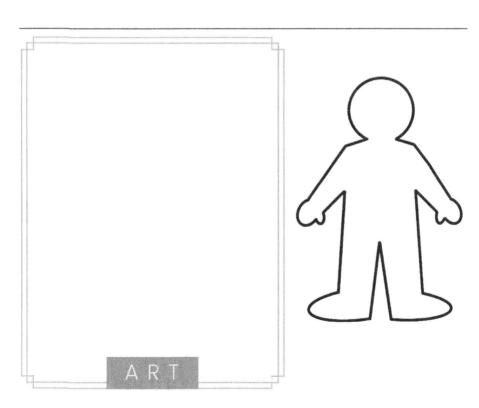

ART

date:_____

Today, I feel_____

about _____

_____

because_____

_____

I need_____

_____

I choose_____

_____

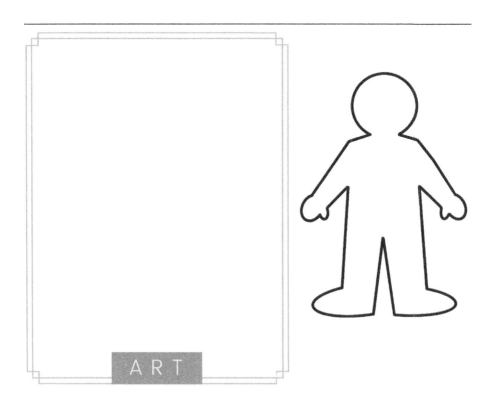

ART

date:_____

Today, I feel_____

about _____

_____

because_____

_____

I need_____

_____

I choose_____

_____

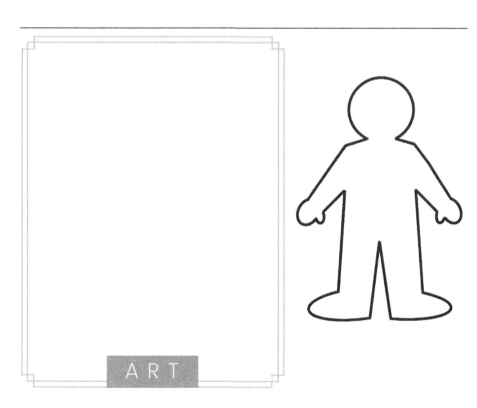

A R T

date:_____

Today, I feel_____

about _____

_____

because_____

_____

I need_____

_____

I choose _____

_____

ART

date:_____

Today, I feel_____

about _____

_____

because_____

_____

I need_____

_____

I choose _____

_____

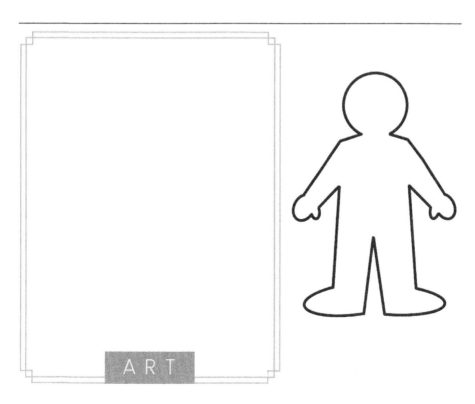

ART

date:_____

Today, I feel_____

about _____
_____

because_____
_____

I need_____
_____

I choose _____
_____

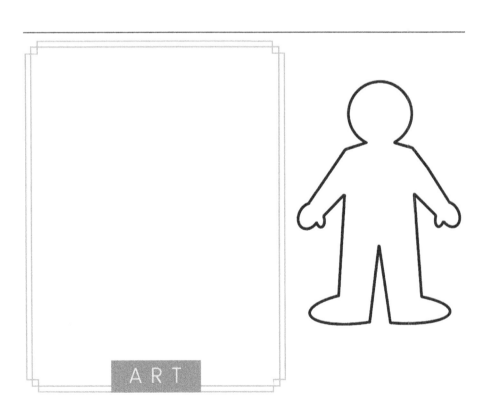

ART

date:_____

Today, I feel_____

about _____

_____

because_____

_____

I need_____

_____

I choose _____

_____

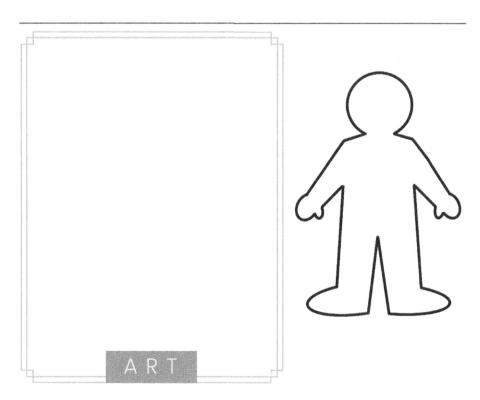

ART

date:_____

Today, I feel_____

about _____

_____

because_____

_____

I need_____

_____

I choose_____

_____

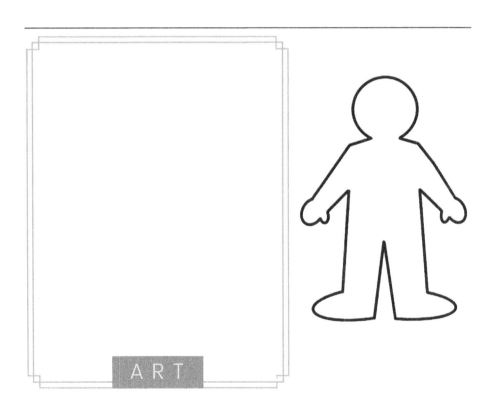

ART

date:_____

Today, I feel_____

about _____

_____

because_____

_____

I need_____

_____

I choose _____

_____

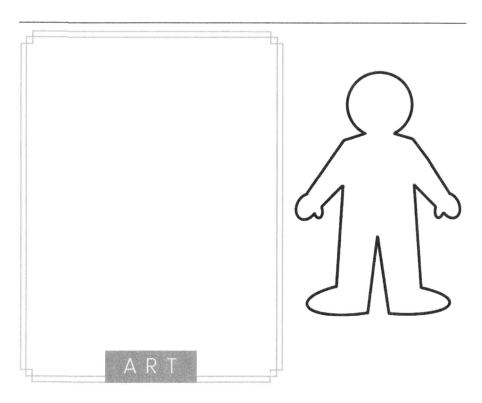

A R T

date:_____

Today, I feel_____

about _____

_____

because_____

_____

I need_____

_____

I choose_____

_____

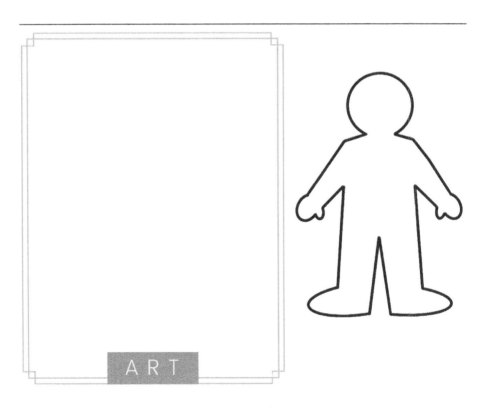

ART

date:_____

Today, I feel_____

about _____

_____

because_____

_____

I need_____

_____

I choose_____

_____

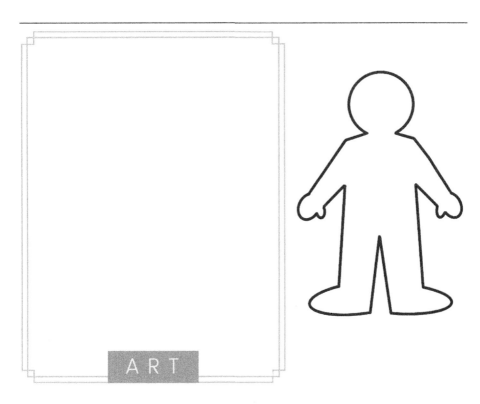

A R T

date:_____

Today, I feel_____

about _____

_____

because_____

_____

I need_____

_____

I choose_____

_____

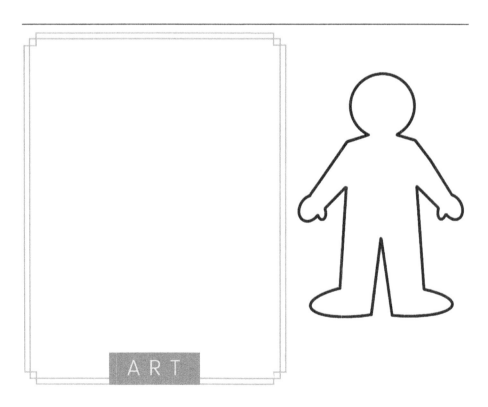

ART

date:_____

Today, I feel_____

about _____

_____

because_____

_____

I need_____

_____

I choose _____

_____

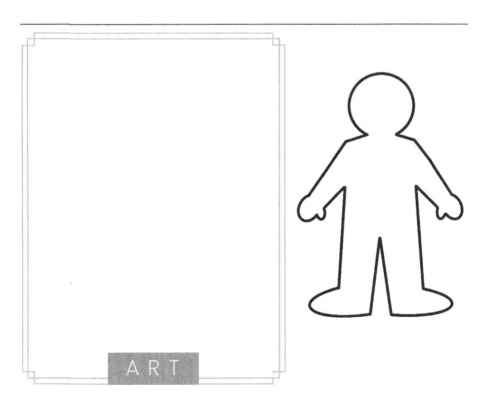

ART

date:_____

Today, I feel_____

about _____

_____

because_____

_____

I need_____

_____

I choose_____

_____

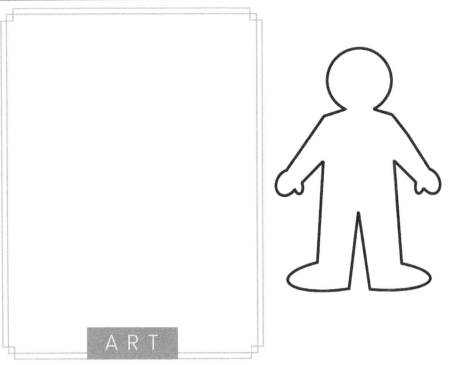

ART

date:_____

Today, I feel_____

about _____

_____

because_____

_____

I need_____

_____

I choose _____

_____

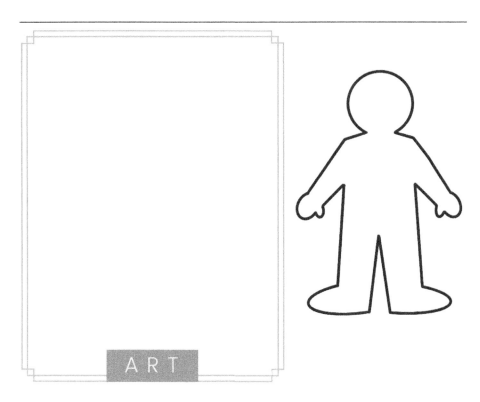

ART

date:_____

Today, I feel_____

about _____

_____

because_____

_____

I need_____

_____

I choose_____

_____

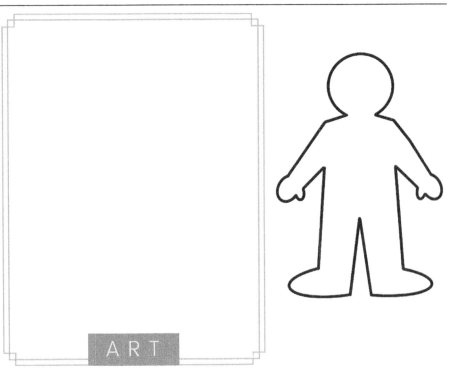

ART

date:_____

Today, I feel_____

about _____

_____

because_____

_____

I need_____

_____

I choose_____

_____

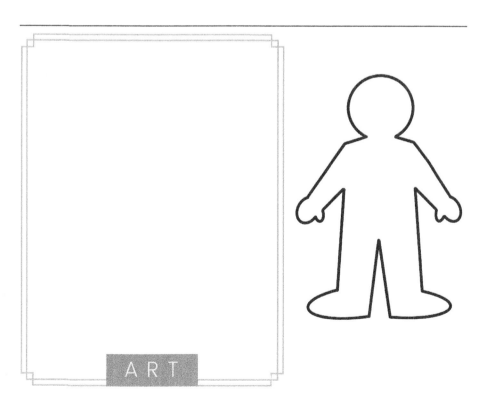

ART

date:_____

Today, I feel_____

about _____

_____

because_____

_____

I need_____

_____

I choose _____

_____

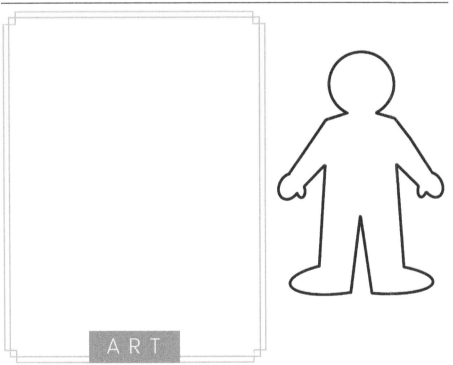

ART

date:_____

Today, I feel_____

about _____

_____

because_____

_____

I need_____

_____

I choose _____

_____

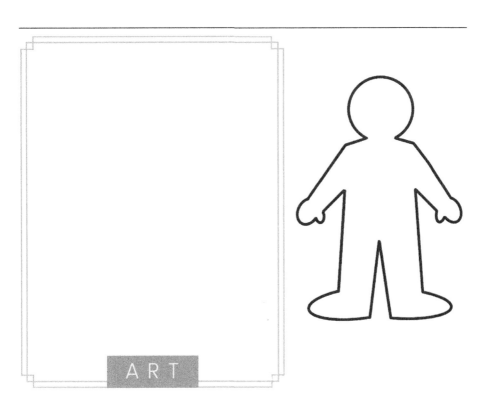

ART

date:_____

Today, I feel_____

about _____

_____

because_____

_____

I need_____

_____

I choose_____

_____

ART

date:_____

Today, I feel_____

about _____

_____

because_____

_____

I need_____

_____

I choose_____

_____

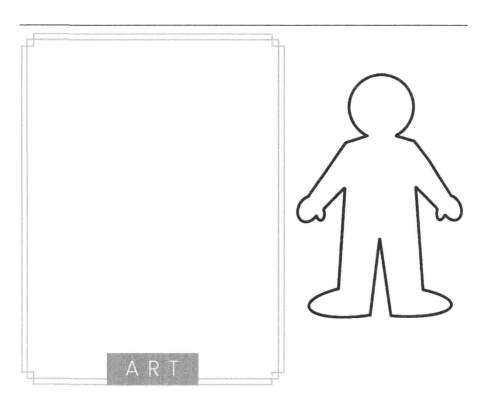

ART

date:_____

Today, I feel_____

about _____

_____

because_____

_____

I need_____

_____

I choose_____

_____

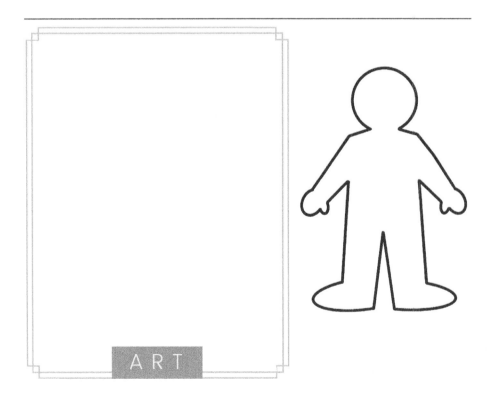

ART

date:_____

Today, I feel_____

about _____

_____

because_____

_____

I need_____

_____

I choose _____

_____

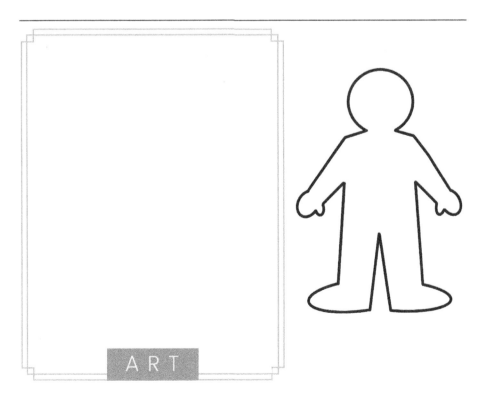

ART

date:_____

Today, I feel_____

about _____

_____

because_____

_____

I need_____

_____

I choose_____

_____

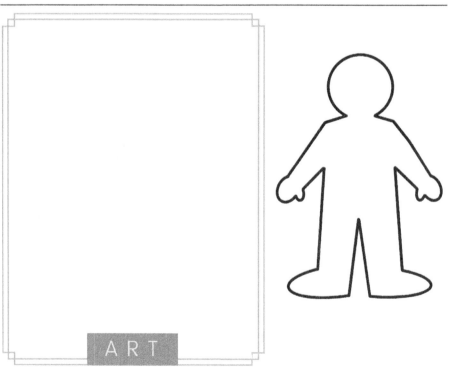

ART

date:_____

Today, I feel_____

about _____

_____

because_____

_____

I need_____

_____

I choose _____

_____

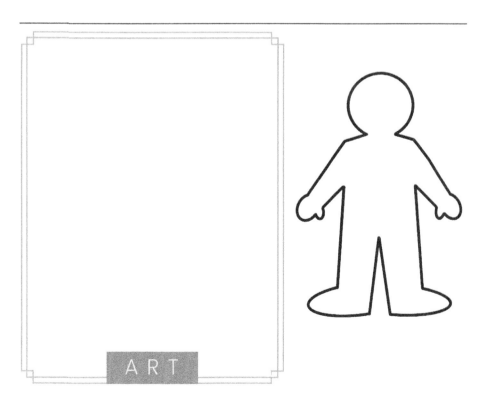

ART

date:_____

Today, I feel_____

about _____

_____

because_____

_____

I need_____

_____

I choose_____

_____

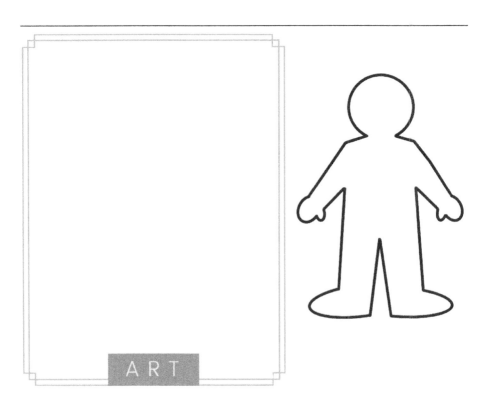

ART

date:_____

Today, I feel_____

about _____

_____

because_____

_____

I need_____

_____

I choose_____

_____

A R T

date:_____

Today, I feel_____

about _____

_____

because_____

_____

I need_____

_____

I choose_____

_____

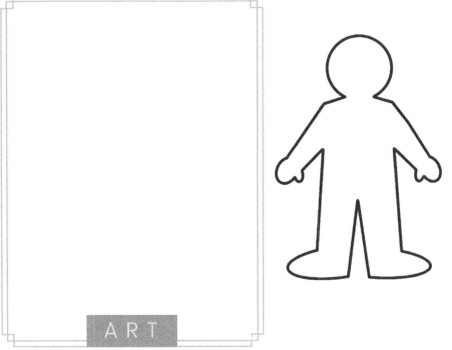

ART

date:_____

Today, I feel_____

about _____

_____

because_____

_____

I need_____

_____

I choose _____

_____

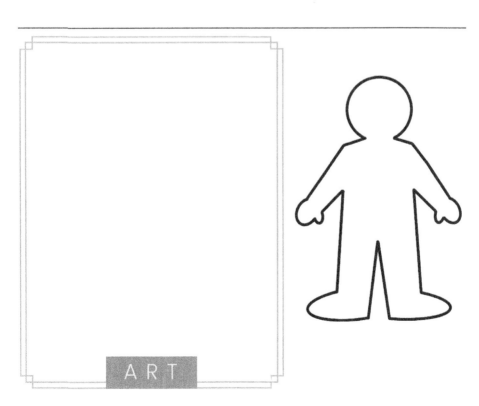

ART

date:_____

Today, I feel_____

about _____

_____

because_____

_____

I need_____

_____

I choose_____

_____

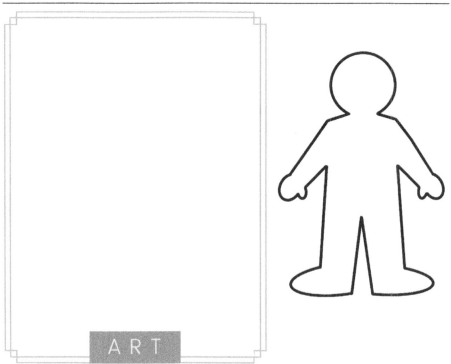

ART

date:_____

Today, I feel_____

about _____

_____

because_____

_____

I need_____

_____

I choose_____

_____

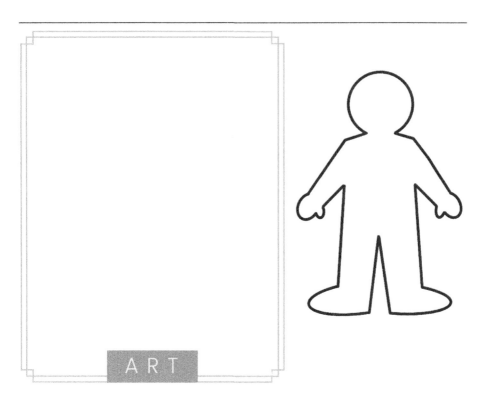

ART

date:_____

Today, I feel_____

about _____

_____

because_____

_____

I need_____

_____

I choose_____

_____

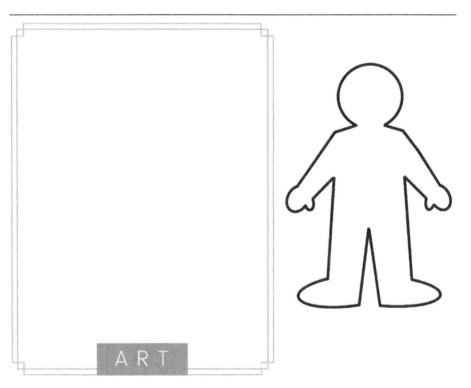

ART

date:_____

Today, I feel_____

about _____

_____

because_____

_____

I need_____

_____

I choose _____

_____

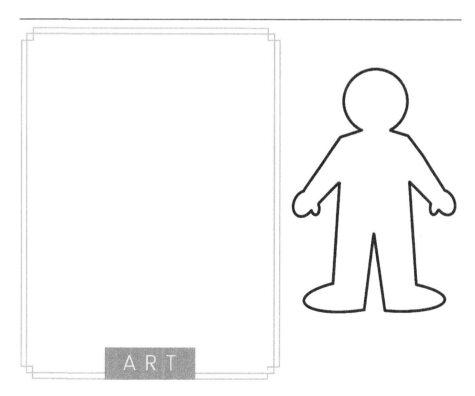

ART

date:_____

Today, I feel_____

about _____

_____

because_____

_____

I need_____

_____

I choose_____

_____

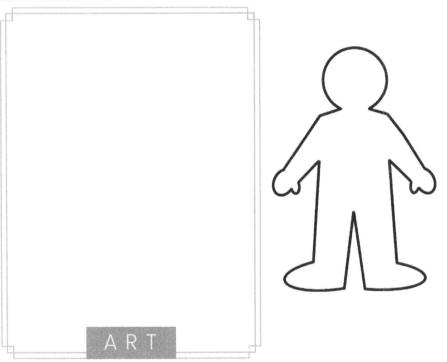

ART

date:_____

Today, I feel_____

about _____

_____

because_____

_____

I need_____

_____

I choose _____

_____

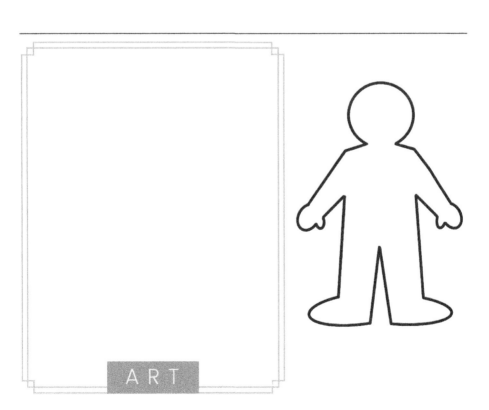

ART

date:_____

Today, I feel_____

about _____

_____

because_____

_____

I need_____

_____

I choose_____

_____

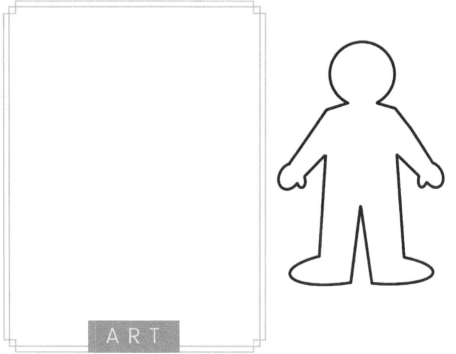

ART

date:_____

Today, I feel_____

about _____

_____

because_____

_____

I need_____

_____

I choose _____

_____

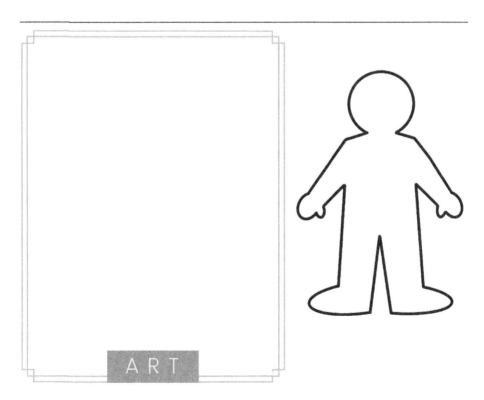

ART

date:_____

Today, I feel_____

about _____

_____

because_____

_____

I need_____

_____

I choose _____

_____

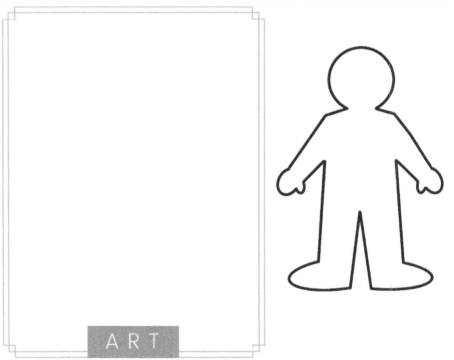

ART

date:_____

Today, I feel_____

about _____

_____

because_____

_____

I need_____

_____

I choose_____

_____

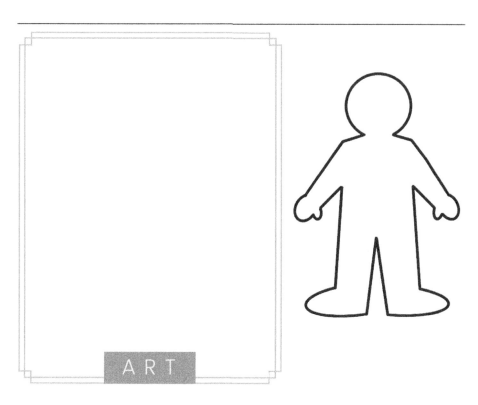

ART

date:_____

Today, I feel_____

about _____

_____

because_____

_____

I need_____

_____

I choose _____

_____

ART

date:_____

Today, I feel_____

about _____

_____

because_____

_____

I need_____

_____

I choose _____

_____

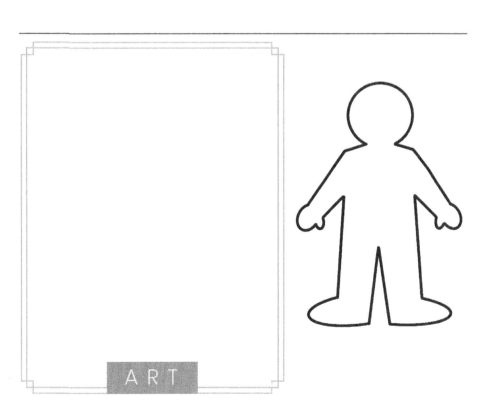

ART

date:_____

Today, I feel_____

about _____

_____

because_____

_____

I need_____

_____

I choose _____

_____

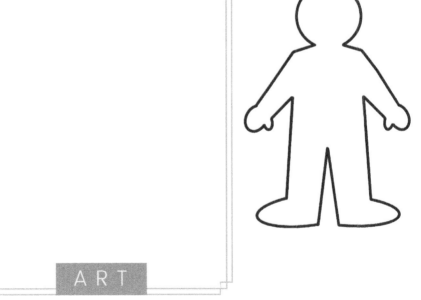

ART

date:_____

Today, I feel_____

about _____

_____

because_____

_____

I need_____

_____

I choose_____

_____

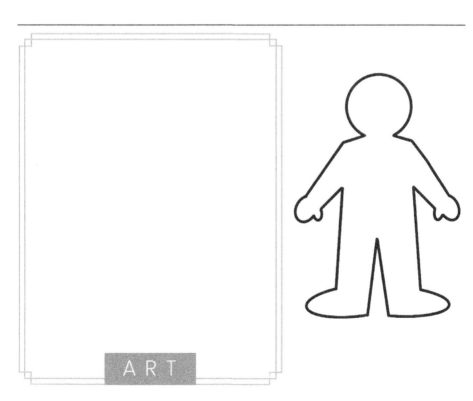

ART

date:_____

Today, I feel_____

about _____

_____

because_____

_____

I need_____

_____

I choose _____

_____

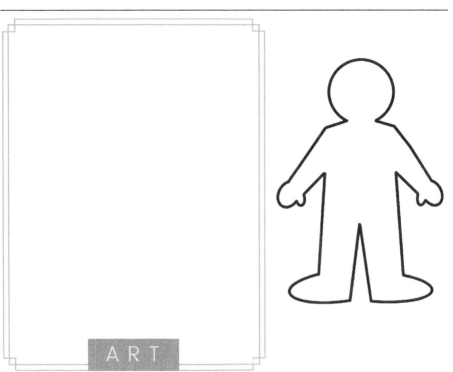

ART

date:_____

Today, I feel_____

about _____

_____

because_____

_____

I need_____

_____

I choose_____

_____

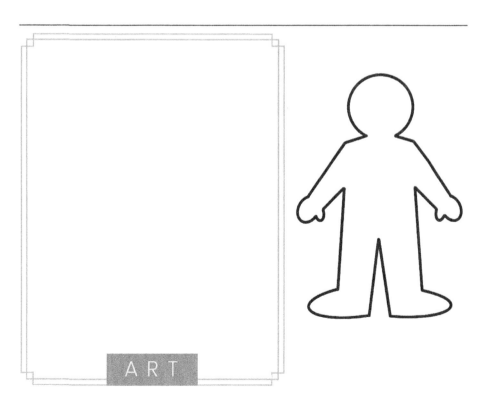

ART

date:_____

Today, I feel_____

about _____

_____

because_____

_____

I need_____

_____

I choose_____

_____

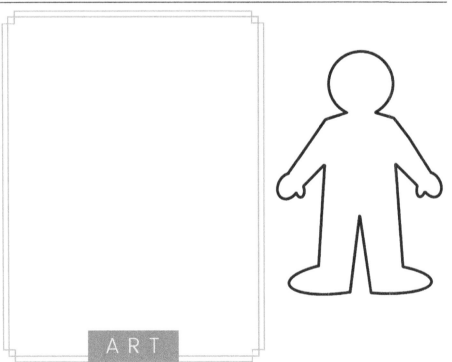

ART

date:_____

Today, I feel_____

about _____

_____

because_____

_____

I need_____

_____

I choose_____

_____

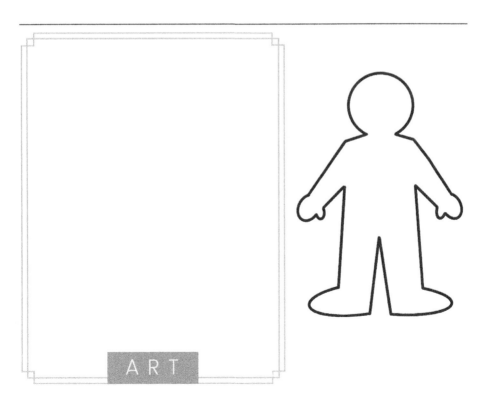

ART

date:_____

Today, I feel_____

about _____

_____

because_____

_____

I need_____

_____

I choose _____

_____

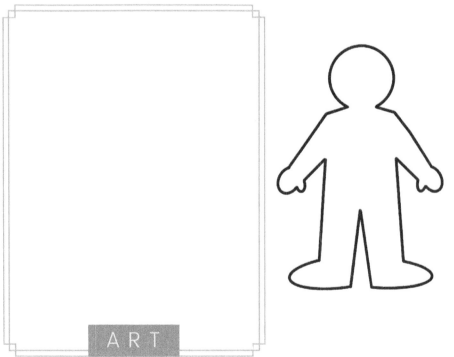

ART

date:_____

Today, I feel_____

about _____

_____

because_____

_____

I need_____

_____

I choose _____

_____

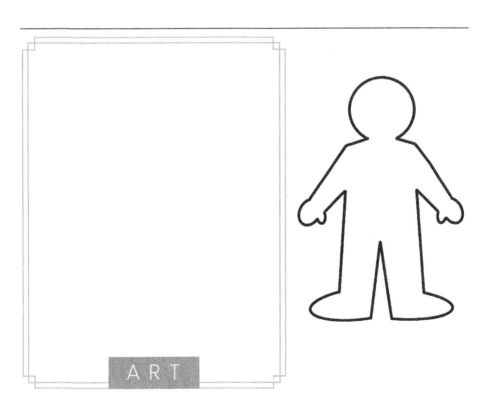

ART

date:_____

Today, I feel_____

about _____

_____

because_____

_____

I need_____

_____

I choose_____

_____

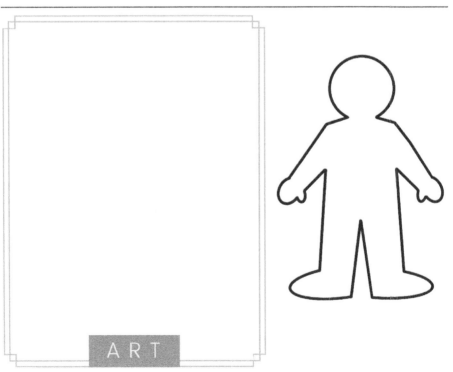

ART

date:_____

Today, I feel_____

about _____

_____

because_____

_____

I need_____

_____

I choose _____

_____

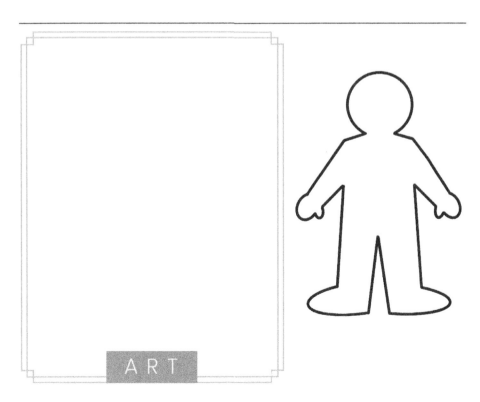

ART

date:_____

Today, I feel_____

about _____

_____

because_____

_____

I need_____

_____

I choose_____

_____

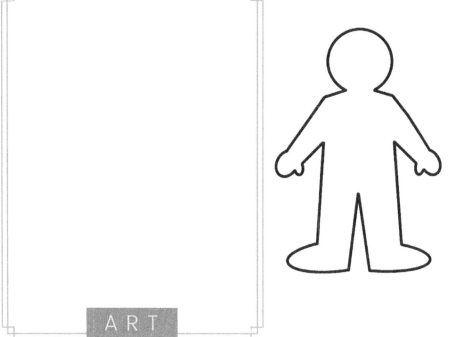

ART

date:_____

Today, I feel_____

about _____

_____

because_____

_____

I need_____

_____

I choose _____

_____

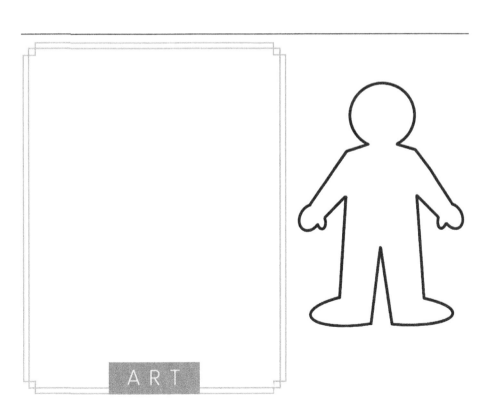

ART

date:_____

Today, I feel_____

about _____

_____

because_____

_____

I need_____

_____

I choose_____

_____

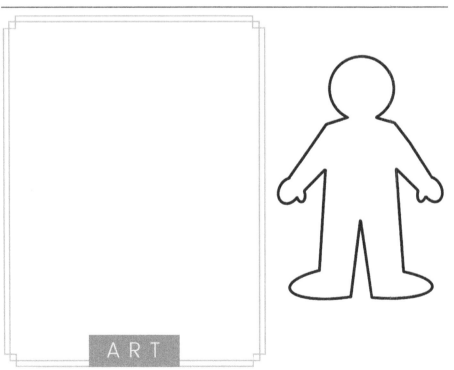

ART

date:_____

Today, I feel_____

about _____

_____

because_____

_____

I need_____

_____

I choose_____

_____

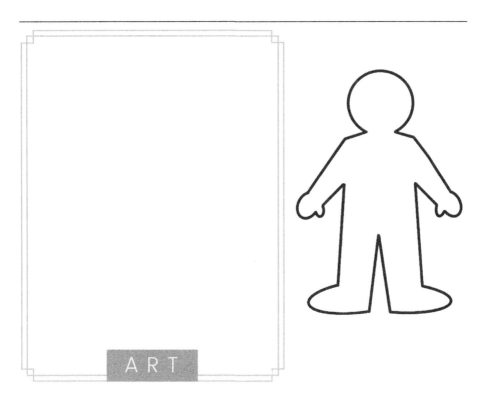

ART

date:_____

Today, I feel_____

about _____

_____

because_____

_____

I need_____

_____

I choose _____

_____

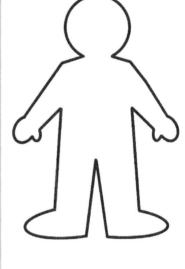

date:_____

Today, I feel_____

about _____

_____

because_____

_____

I need_____

_____

I choose_____

_____

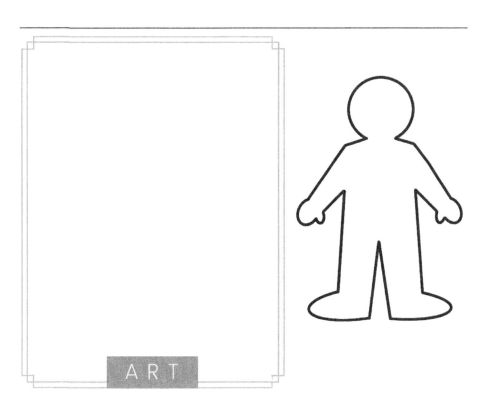

ART

date:_____

Today, I feel_____

about _____

_____

because_____

_____

I need_____

_____

I choose_____

_____

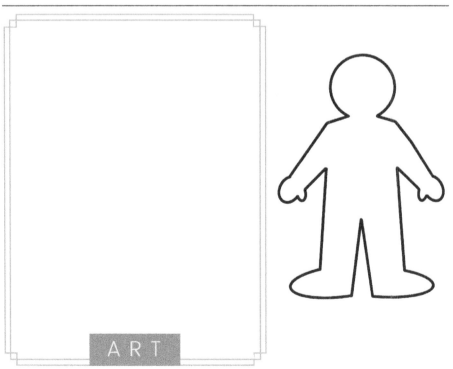

ART

date:_____

Today, I feel_____

about _____

_____

because_____

_____

I need_____

_____

I choose _____

_____

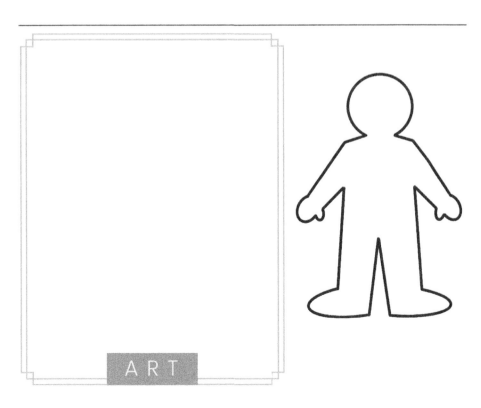

ART

date:_____

Today, I feel_____

about _____

_____

because_____

_____

I need_____

_____

I choose _____

_____

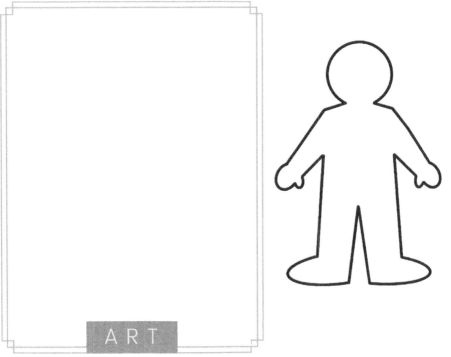

ART

date:_____

Today, I feel_____

about _____

_____

because_____

_____

I need_____

_____

I choose _____

_____

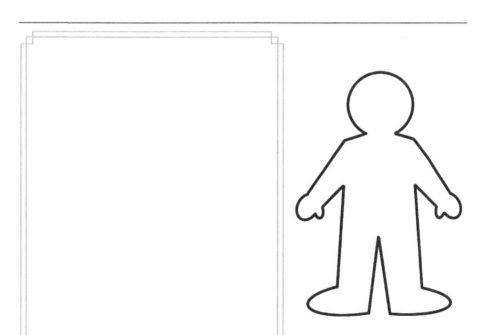

ART

date:_____

Today, I feel_____

about _____

_____

because_____

_____

I need_____

_____

I choose_____

_____

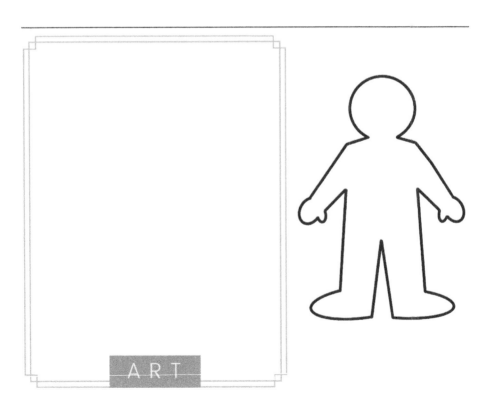

ART

date:_____

Today, I feel_____

about _____

_____

because_____

_____

I need_____

_____

I choose _____

_____

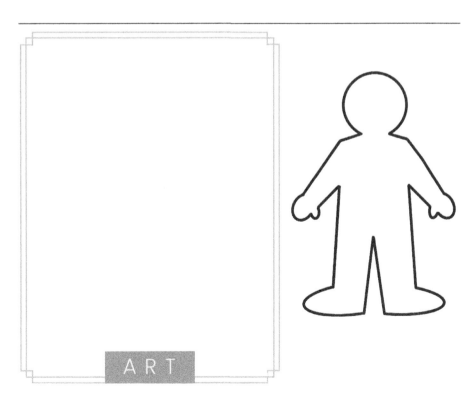

ART

date:_____

Today, I feel_____

about _____

_____

because_____

_____

I need_____

_____

I choose_____

_____

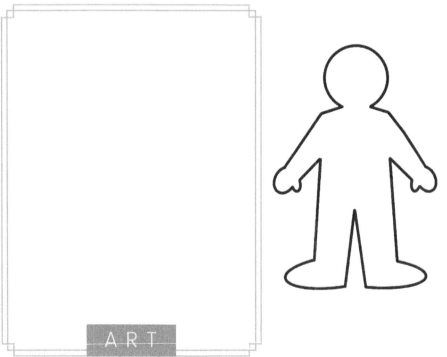

ART

date:_____

Today, I feel_____

about _____

_____

because_____

_____

I need_____

_____

I choose_____

_____

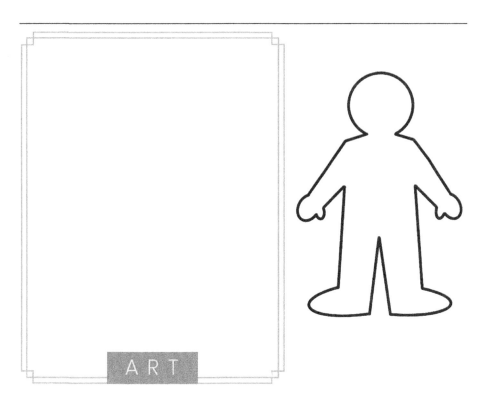

ART

date:_____

Today, I feel_____

about _____

_____

because_____

_____

I need_____

_____

I choose_____

_____

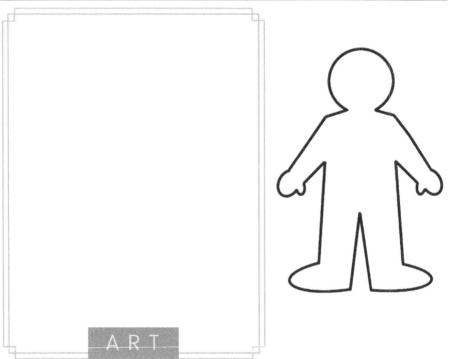

ART

date:_____

Today, I feel_____

about _____

_____

because_____

_____

I need_____

_____

I choose _____

_____

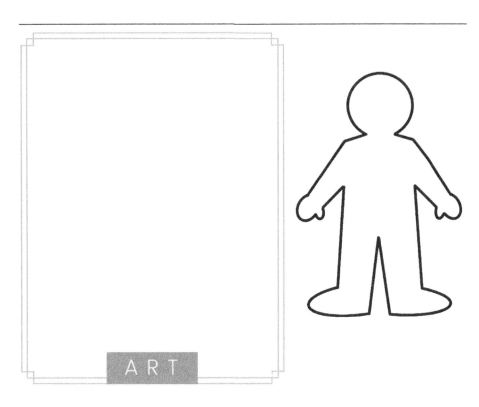

ART

date:_____

Today, I feel_____

about _____

_____

because_____

_____

I need_____

_____

I choose_____

_____

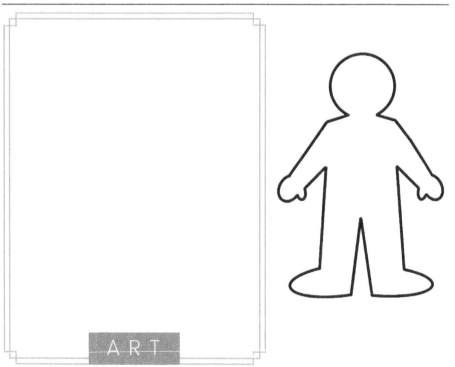

ART

date:_____

Today, I feel_____

about _____

_____

because_____

_____

I need_____

_____

I choose_____

_____

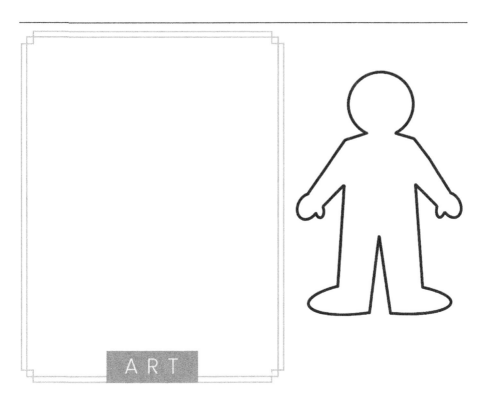

ART

date:_____

Today, I feel_____

about _____

_____

because_____

_____

I need_____

_____

I choose _____

_____

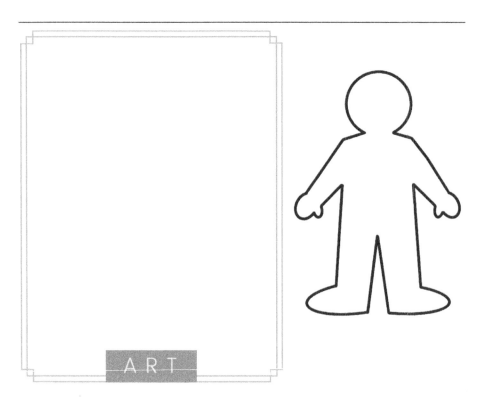

ART

date:_____

Today, I feel_____

about _____

_____

because_____

_____

I need_____

_____

I choose _____

_____

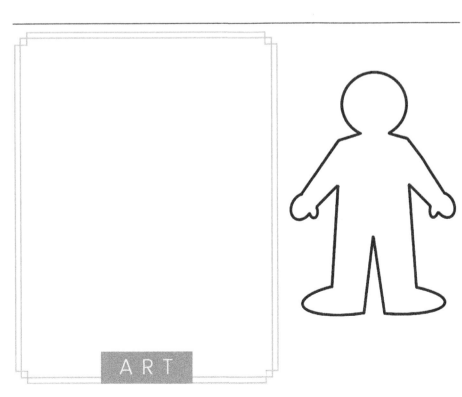

ART

date:_____

Today, I feel_____

about _____

_____

because_____

_____

I need_____

_____

I choose_____

_____

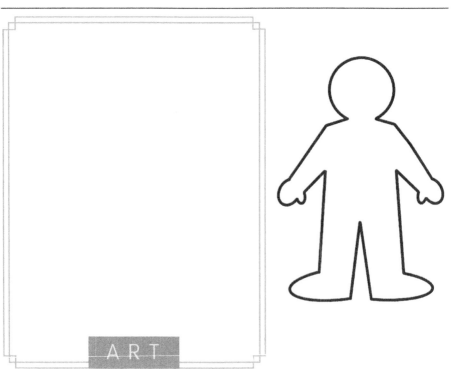

ART

date:_____

Today, I feel_____

about _____

_____

because_____

_____

I need_____

_____

I choose _____

_____

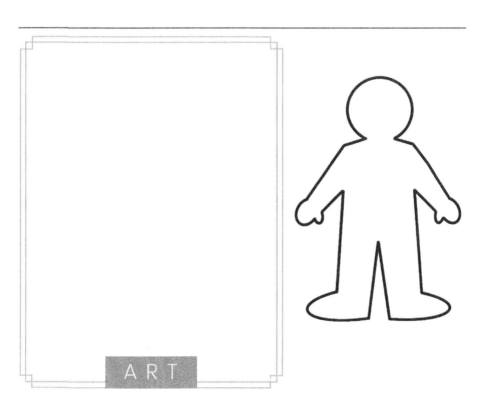

ART

date:_____

Today, I feel_____

about _____

_____

because_____

_____

I need_____

_____

I choose _____

_____

date:_____

Today, I feel_____

about _____

_____

because_____

_____

I need_____

_____

I choose _____

_____

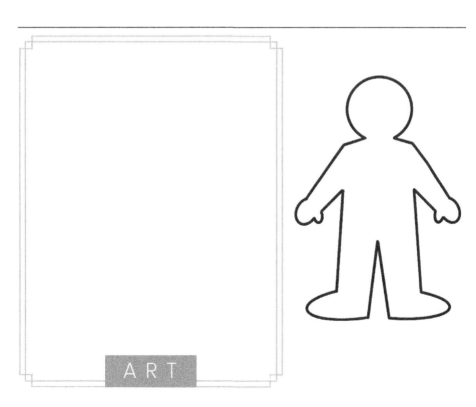

ART

date:_____

Today, I feel_____

about _____

_____

because_____

_____

I need_____

_____

I choose_____

_____

ART

date:_____

Today, I feel_____

about _____

_____

because_____

_____

I need_____

_____

I choose_____

_____

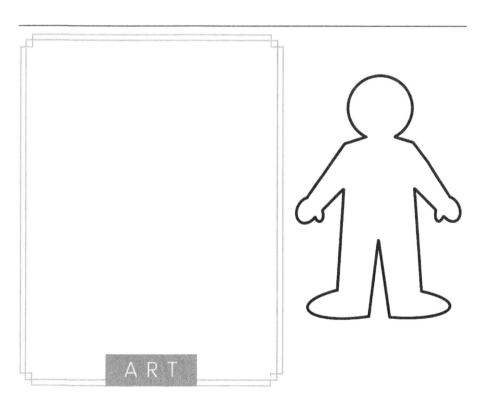

ART

date:_____

Today, I feel_____

about _____

_____

because_____

_____

I need_____

_____

I choose _____

_____

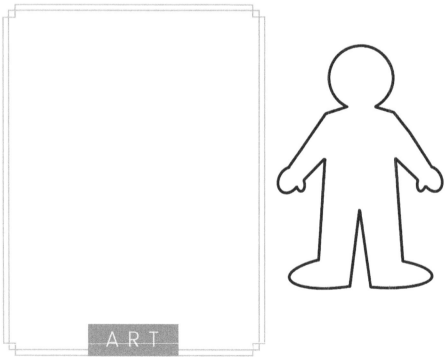

ART

date:_____

Today, I feel_____

about _____

_____

because_____

_____

I need_____

_____

I choose _____

_____

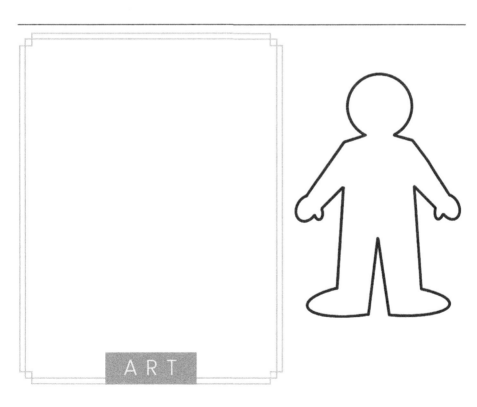

ART

date:_____

Today, I feel_____

about _____

_____

because_____

_____

I need_____

_____

I choose_____

_____

ART

date:_____

Today, I feel_____

about _____

_____

because_____

_____

I need_____

_____

I choose _____

_____

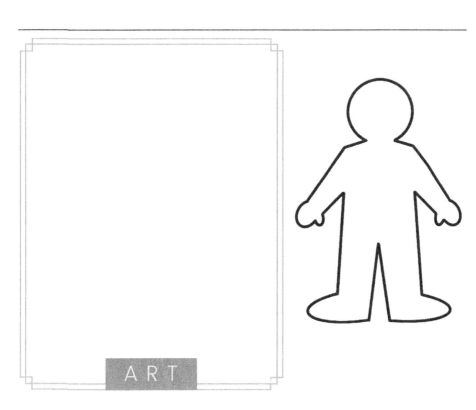

A R T

date:_____

Today, I feel_____

about _____

_____

because_____

_____

I need_____

_____

I choose _____

_____

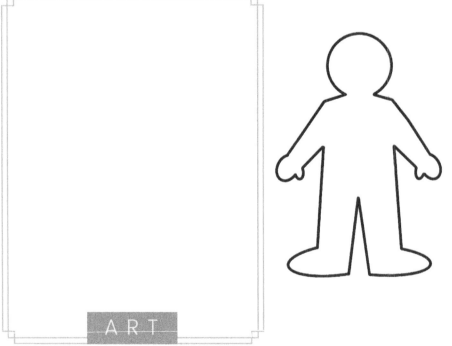

A R T

date:_____

Today, I feel_____

about _____

_____

because_____

_____

I need_____

_____

I choose _____

_____

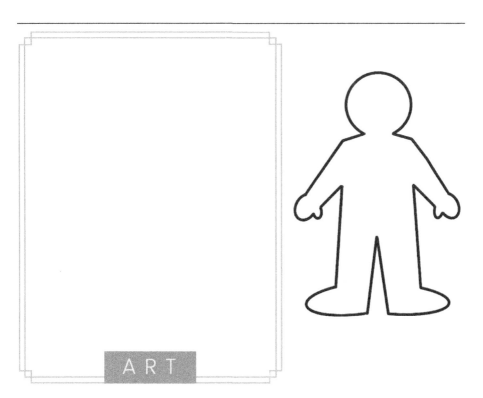

ART

date:_____

Today, I feel_____

about _____

_____

because_____

_____

I need_____

_____

I choose_____

_____

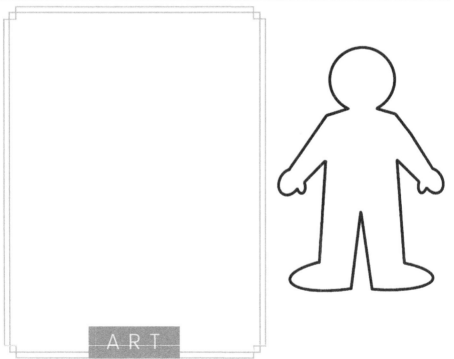

ART

date:_____

Today, I feel_____

about _____

_____

because_____

_____

I need_____

_____

I choose _____

_____

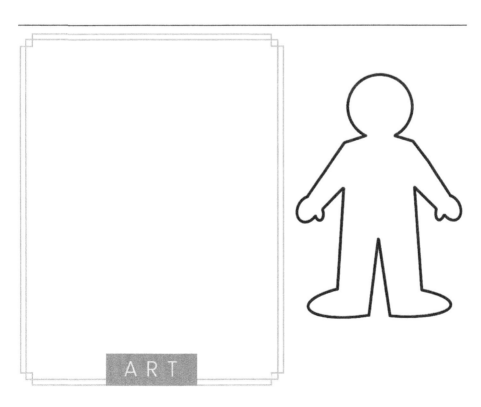

ART

date:_____

Today, I feel_____

about _____

_____

because_____

_____

I need_____

_____

I choose_____

_____

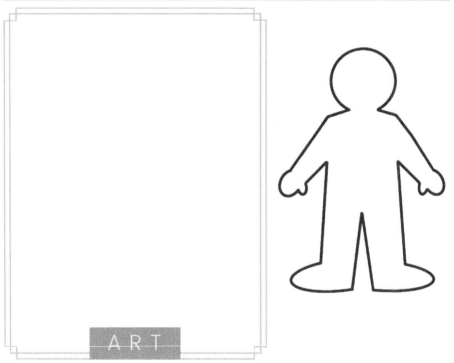

A R T

date:_____

Today, I feel_____

about _____

_____

because_____

_____

I need_____

_____

I choose _____

_____

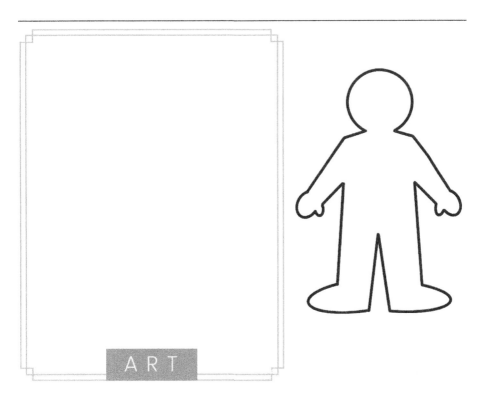

ART

date:_____

Today, I feel_____

about _____

_____

because_____

_____

I need_____

_____

I choose_____

_____

ART

date:_____

Today, I feel_____

about _____

_____

because_____

_____

I need_____

_____

I choose _____

_____

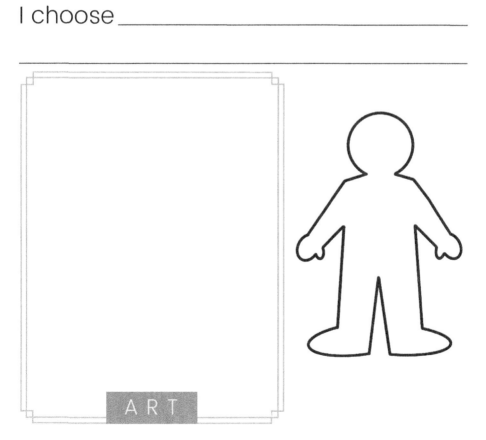

ART

date:_____

Today, I feel_____

about _____

_____

because_____

_____

I need_____

_____

I choose _____

_____

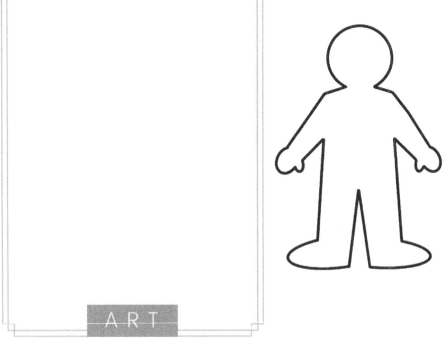

ART

date:_____

Today, I feel_____

about _____

_____

because_____

_____

I need_____

_____

I choose _____

_____

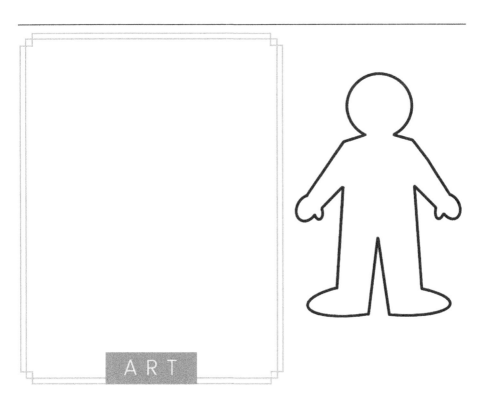

ART

date:_____

Today, I feel_____

about _____

_____

because_____

_____

I need_____

_____

I choose_____

_____

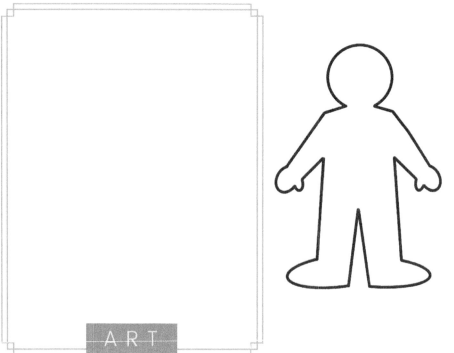

ART

date:_____

Today, I feel_____

about _____

_____

because_____

_____

I need_____

_____

I choose _____

_____

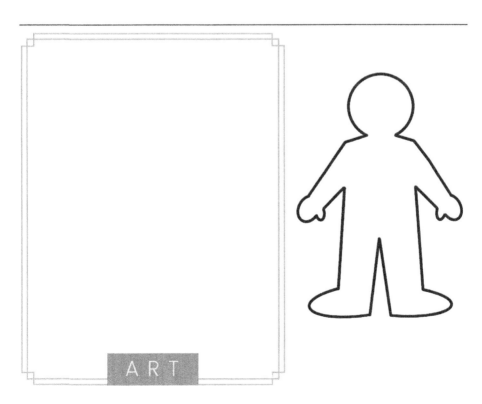

ART

date:_____

Today, I feel_____

about _____

_____

because_____

_____

I need_____

_____

I choose _____

_____

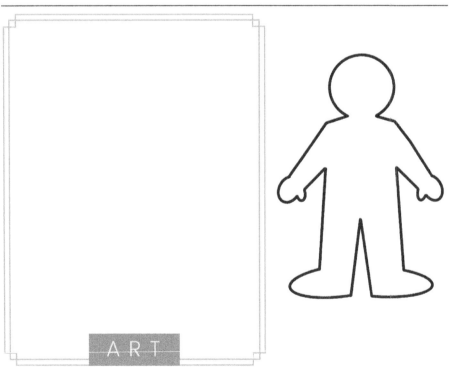

ART

date:_____

Today, I feel_____

about _____

_____

because_____

_____

I need_____

_____

I choose_____

_____

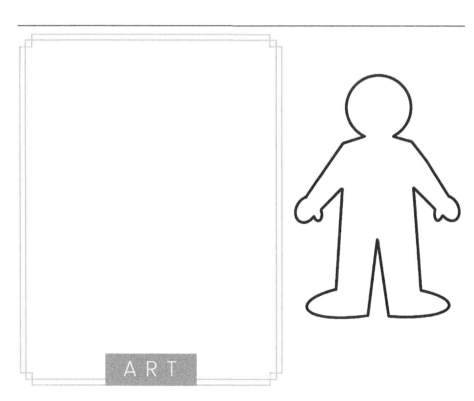

ART

date:_____

Today, I feel_____

about _____

_____

because_____

_____

I need_____

_____

I choose_____

_____

A R T

date:_____

Today, I feel_____

about _____

_____

because_____

_____

I need_____

_____

I choose _____

_____

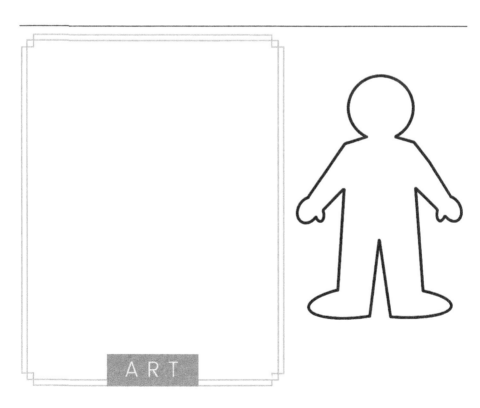

ART

date:_____

Today, I feel_____

about _____

_____

because_____

_____

I need_____

_____

I choose_____

_____

ART

date:_____

Today, I feel_____

about _____
_____

because_____
_____

I need_____
_____

I choose _____
_____

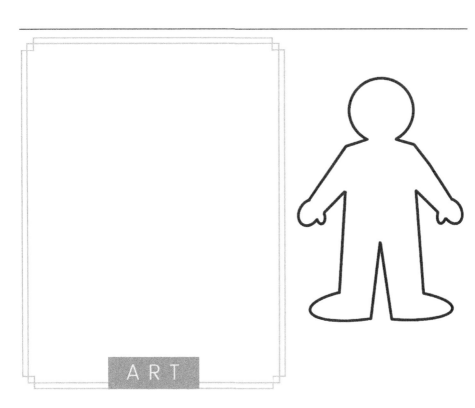

ART

date:_____

Today, I feel_____

about _____

_____

because_____

_____

I need_____

_____

I choose _____

_____

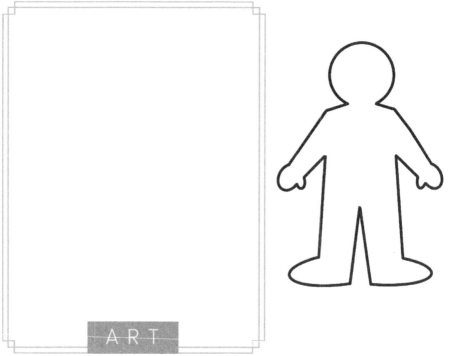

ART

date:_____

Today, I feel_____

about _____

_____

because_____

_____

I need_____

_____

I choose_____

_____

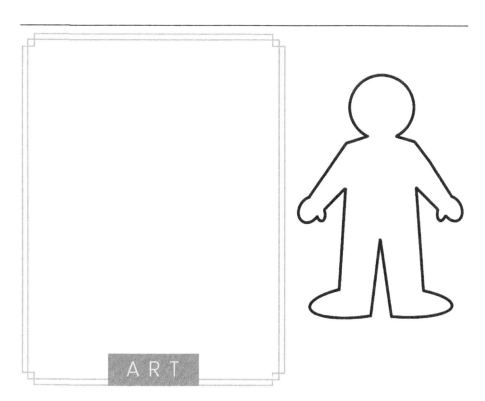

ART

date:_____

Today, I feel_____

about _____

_____

because_____

_____

I need_____

_____

I choose _____

_____

ART

date:_____

Today, I feel_____

about _____

_____

because_____

_____

I need_____

_____

I choose _____

_____

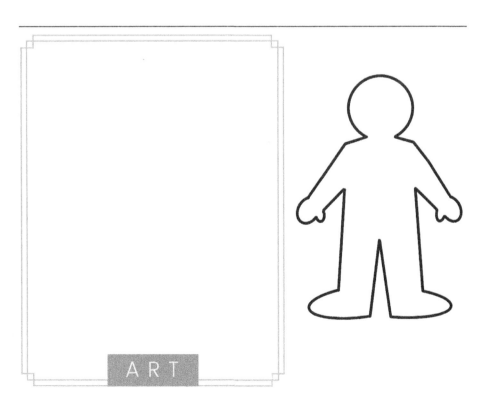

ART

date:_____

Today, I feel_____

about _____

_____

because_____

_____

I need_____

_____

I choose_____

_____

ART

date:_____

Today, I feel_____

about _____
_____

because_____
_____

I need_____
_____

I choose _____
_____

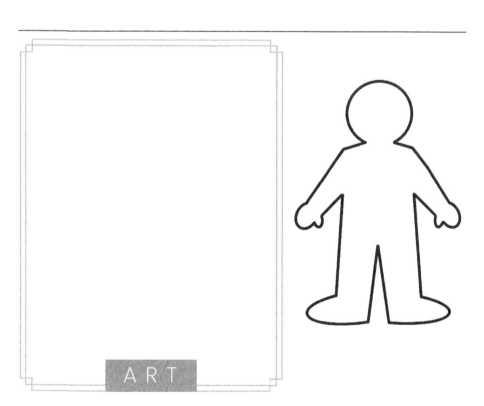

ART

date:_____

Today, I feel_____

about _____

_____

because_____

_____

I need_____

_____

I choose_____

_____

ART

date:_____

Today, I feel_____

about _____
_____

because_____
_____

I need_____
_____

I choose _____
_____

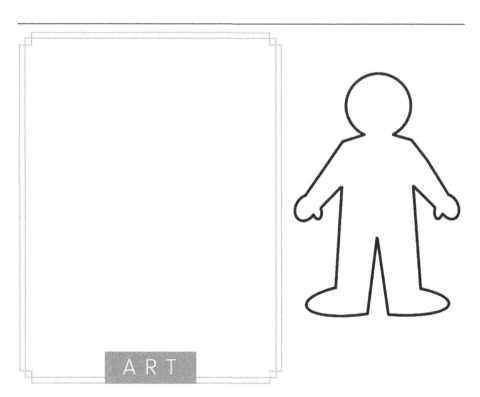

ART

date:_____

Today, I feel_____

about _____

_____

because_____

_____

I need_____

_____

I choose_____

_____

ART

date:_____

Today, I feel_____

about _____

_____

because_____

_____

I need_____

_____

I choose _____

_____

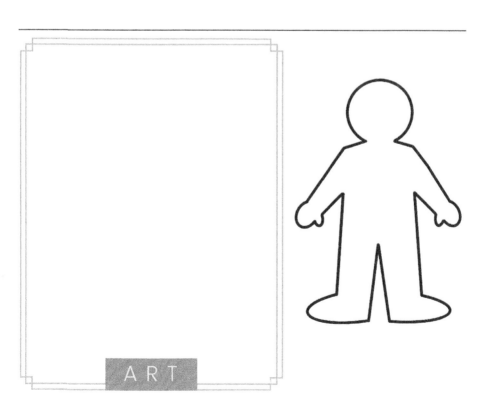

ART

date:_____

Today, I feel_____

about _____

_____

because_____

_____

I need_____

_____

I choose _____

_____

ART

date:_____

Today, I feel_____

about _____

_____

because_____

_____

I need_____

_____

I choose _____

_____

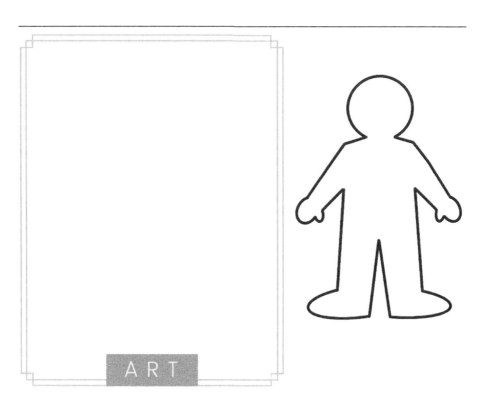

ART

date:_____

Today, I feel_____

about _____

_____

because_____

_____

I need_____

_____

I choose _____

_____

ART

date:_____

Today, I feel_____

about _____
_____

because_____
_____

I need_____
_____

I choose _____
_____

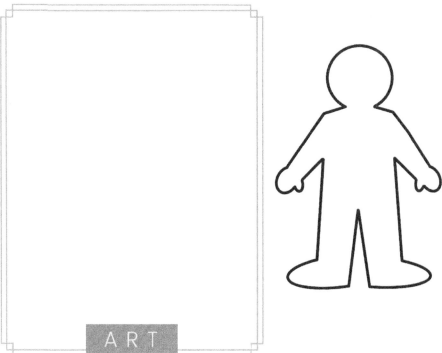

ART

date:_____

Today, I feel_____

about _____

_____

because_____

_____

I need_____

_____

I choose_____

_____

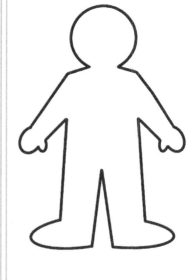

date:_____

Today, I feel_____

about _____

_____

because_____

_____

I need_____

_____

I choose _____

_____

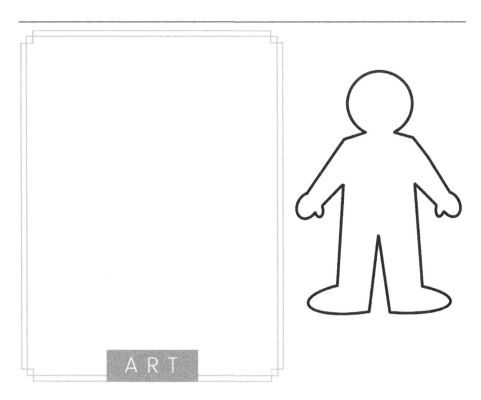

ART

date:_____

Today, I feel_____

about _____

_____

because_____

_____

I need_____

_____

I choose_____

_____

ART

date:_____

Today, I feel_____

about _____
_____

because_____
_____

I need_____
_____

I choose _____
_____

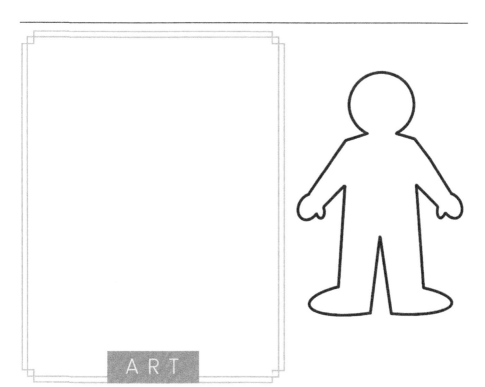

ART

date:_____

Today, I feel_____

about _____

_____

because_____

_____

I need_____

_____

I choose_____

_____

ART

date:_____

Today, I feel_____

about _____

_____

because_____

_____

I need_____

_____

I choose _____

_____

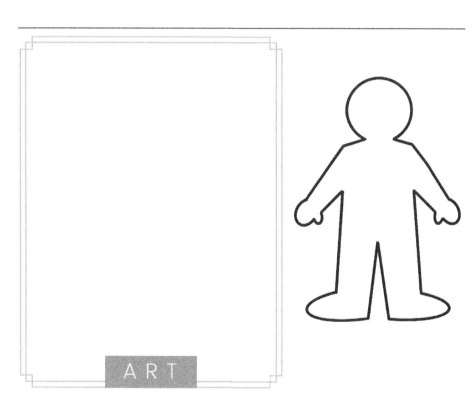

ART

date:_____

Today, I feel_____

about _____

_____

because_____

_____

I need_____

_____

I choose_____

_____

ART

date:_____

Today, I feel_____

about _____

_____

because_____

_____

I need_____

_____

I choose _____

_____

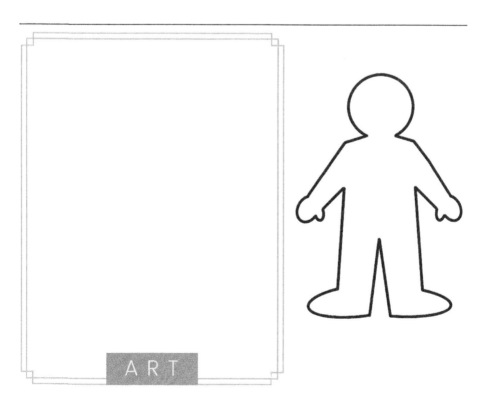

ART

date:_____

Today, I feel_____

about _____

_____

because_____

_____

I need_____

_____

I choose _____

_____

ART

date:_____

Today, I feel_____

about _____

_____

because_____

_____

I need_____

_____

I choose _____

_____

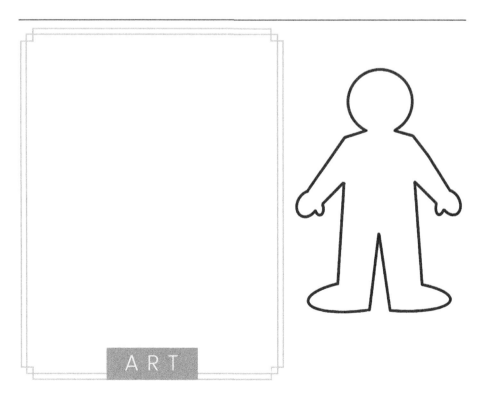

ART

date:_____

Today, I feel_____

about _____

_____

because_____

_____

I need_____

_____

I choose_____

_____

ART

date:_____

Today, I feel_____

about _____

_____

because_____

_____

I need_____

_____

I choose _____

_____

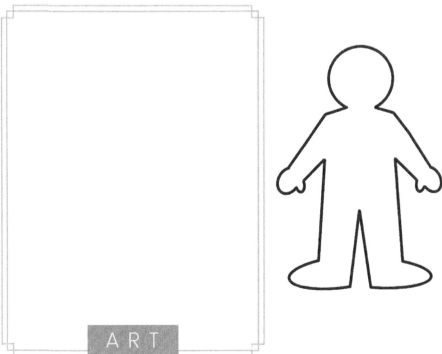

ART

date:_____

Today, I feel_____

about _____

_____

because_____

_____

I need_____

_____

I choose _____

_____

ART

date:_____

Today, I feel_____

about _____

_____

because_____

_____

I need_____

_____

I choose _____

_____

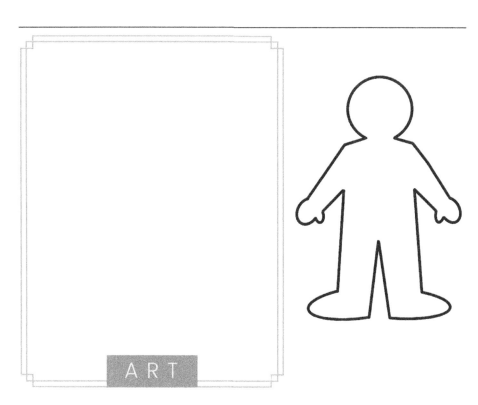

ART

date:_____

Today, I feel_____

about _____

_____

because_____

_____

I need_____

_____

I choose_____

_____

ART

date:_____

Today, I feel_____

about _____

_____

because_____

_____

I need_____

_____

I choose _____

_____

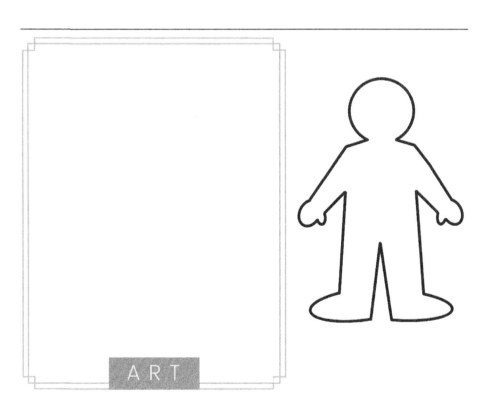

ART

date:_____

Today, I feel_____

about _____

_____

because_____

_____

I need_____

_____

I choose _____

_____

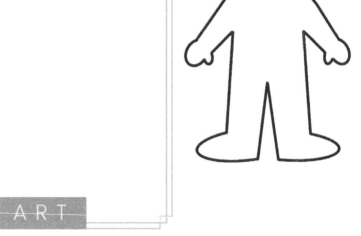

ART

date:_____

Today, I feel_____

about _____

_____

because_____

_____

I need_____

_____

I choose _____

_____

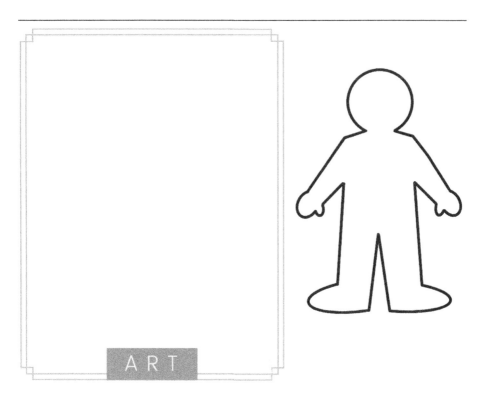

ART

date:_____

Today, I feel_____

about _____

_____

because_____

_____

I need_____

_____

I choose _____

_____

ART

date:_____

Today, I feel_____

about _____

_____

because_____

_____

I need_____

_____

I choose _____

_____

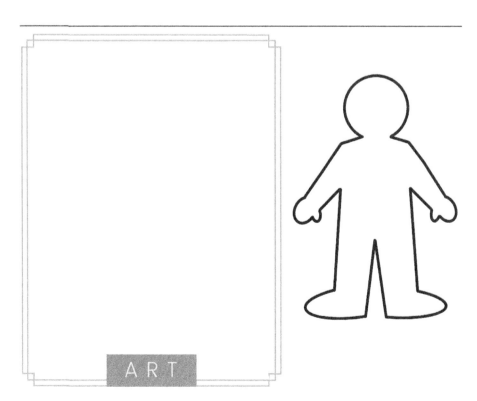

ART

date:_____

Today, I feel_____

about _____

_____

because_____

_____

I need_____

_____

I choose _____

_____

ART

date:_____

Today, I feel_____

about _____

_____

because_____

_____

I need_____

_____

I choose _____

_____

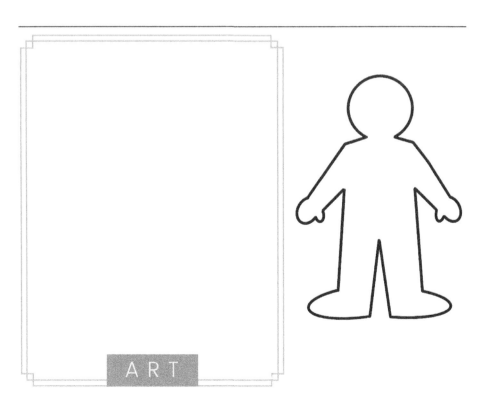

ART

date:_____

Today, I feel_____

about _____

_____

because_____

_____

I need_____

_____

I choose_____

_____

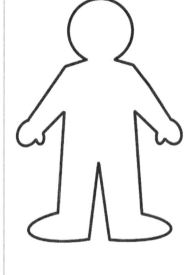

date:_____

Today, I feel_____

about _____
_____

because_____
_____

I need_____
_____

I choose _____
_____

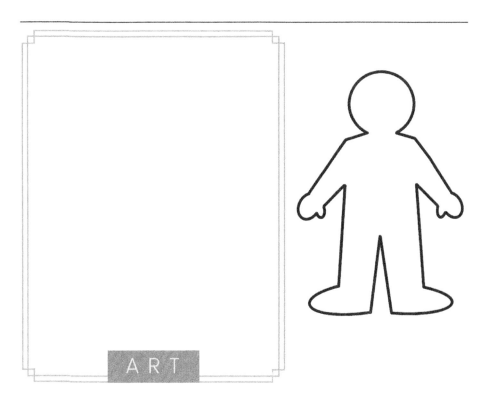

ART

date:_____

Today, I feel_____

about _____

_____

because_____

_____

I need_____

_____

I choose _____

_____

ART

date:_____

Today, I feel_____

about _____

_____

because_____

_____

I need_____

_____

I choose _____

_____

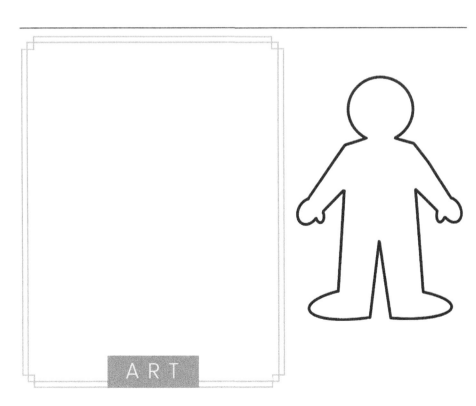

ART

date:_____

Today, I feel_____

about _____

_____

because_____

_____

I need_____

_____

I choose_____

_____

ART

date:_____

Today, I feel_____

about _____
_____

because_____
_____

I need_____
_____

I choose _____
_____

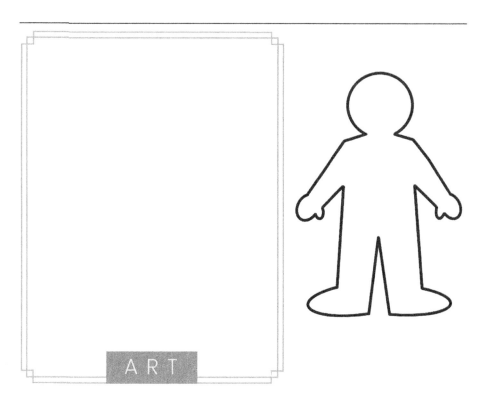

ART

date:_____

Today, I feel_____

about _____

_____

because_____

_____

I need_____

_____

I choose _____

_____

ART

date:_____

Today, I feel_____

about _____

_____

because_____

_____

I need_____

_____

I choose _____

_____

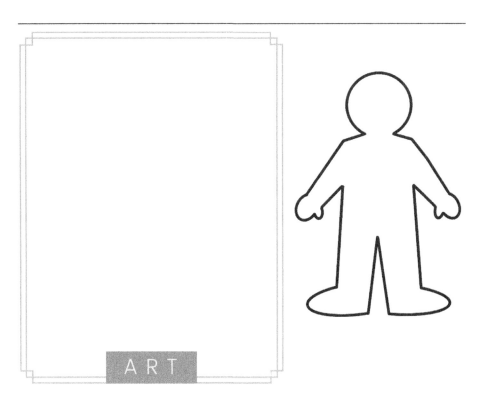

ART

date:_____

Today, I feel_____

about _____

_____

because_____

_____

I need_____

_____

I choose _____

_____

ART

date:_____

Today, I feel_____

about _____

_____

because_____

_____

I need_____

_____

I choose _____

_____

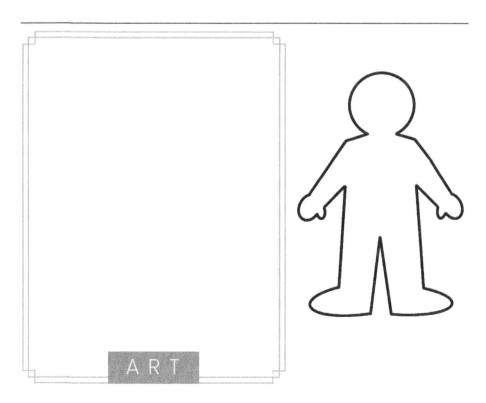

ART

date:_____

Today, I feel_____

about _____

_____

because_____

_____

I need_____

_____

I choose_____

_____

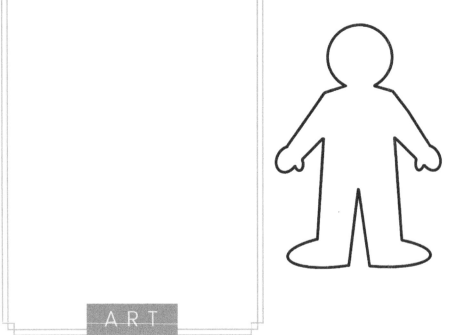

ART

date:_____

Today, I feel_____

about _____

_____

because_____

_____

I need_____

_____

I choose _____

_____

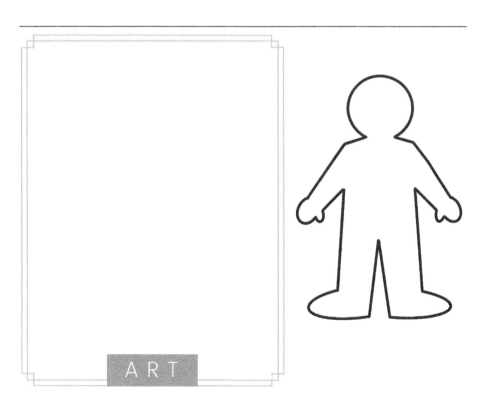

ART

date:_____

Today, I feel_____

about _____

_____

because_____

_____

I need_____

_____

I choose _____

_____

ART

date:_____

Today, I feel_____

about _____

_____

because_____

_____

I need_____

_____

I choose_____

_____

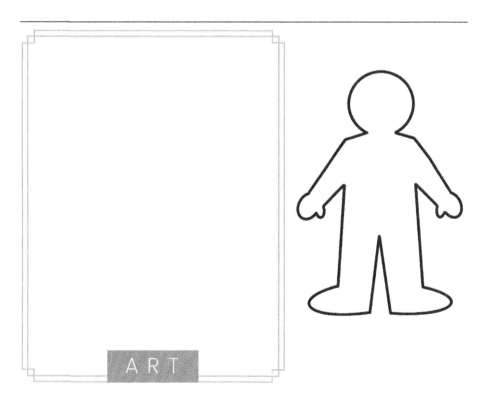

ART

date:_____

Today, I feel_____

about _____

_____

because_____

_____

I need_____

_____

I choose_____

_____

ART

date:_____

Today, I feel_____

about _____

_____

because_____

_____

I need_____

_____

I choose _____

_____

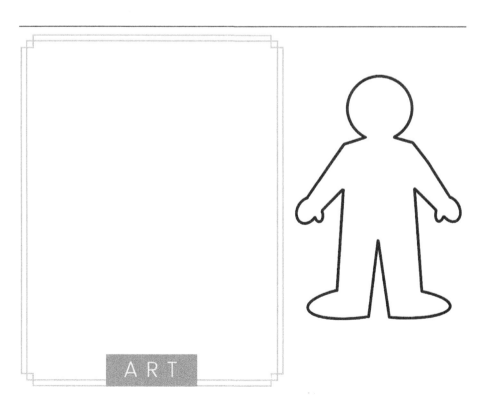

ART

date:_____

Today, I feel_____

about _____

_____

because_____

_____

I need_____

_____

I choose _____

_____

ART

date:_____

Today, I feel_____

about _____

_____

because_____

_____

I need_____

_____

I choose _____

_____

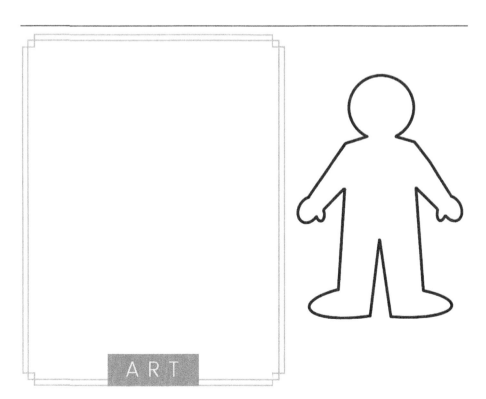

ART

date:_____

Today, I feel_____

about _____

_____

because_____

_____

I need_____

_____

I choose _____

_____

ART

date:_____

Today, I feel_____

about _____

_____

because_____

_____

I need_____

_____

I choose _____

_____

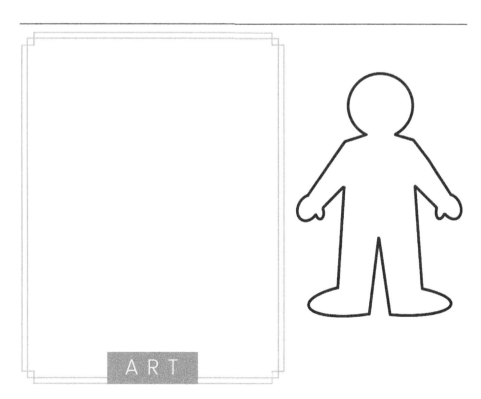

ART

date:_____

Today, I feel_____

about _____

_____

because_____

_____

I need_____

_____

I choose _____

_____

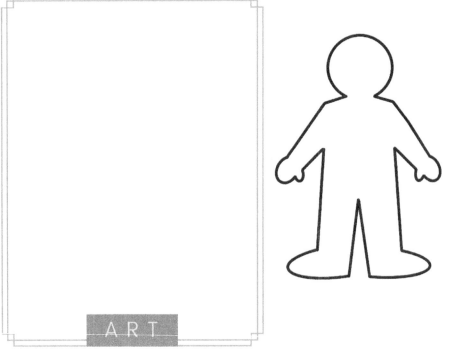

ART

date:_____

Today, I feel_____

about _____

_____

because_____

_____

I need_____

_____

I choose _____

_____

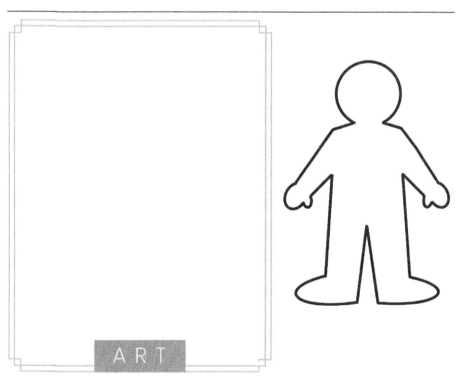

ART

date:_____

Today, I feel_____

about _____

_____

because_____

_____

I need_____

_____

I choose _____

_____

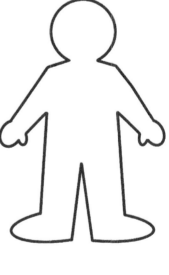

date:_____

Today, I feel_____

about _____

_____

because_____

_____

I need_____

_____

I choose _____

_____

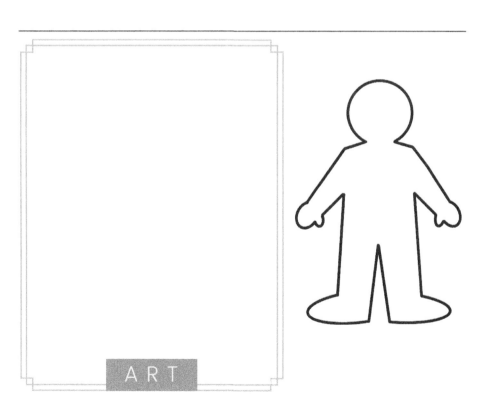

ART

date:_____

Today, I feel_____

about _____

_____

because_____

_____

I need_____

_____

I choose _____

_____

ART

date:_____

Today, I feel_____

about _____

_____

because_____

_____

I need_____

_____

I choose_____

_____

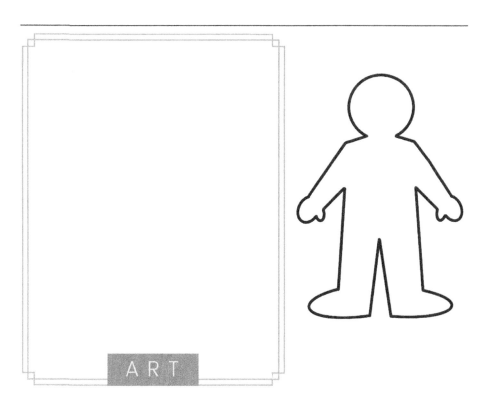

ART

date:_____

Today, I feel_____

about _____

_____

because_____

_____

I need_____

_____

I choose_____

_____

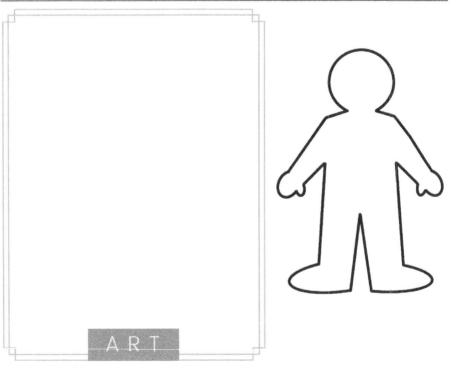

ART

date:_____

Today, I feel_____

about _____

_____

because_____

_____

I need_____

_____

I choose _____

_____

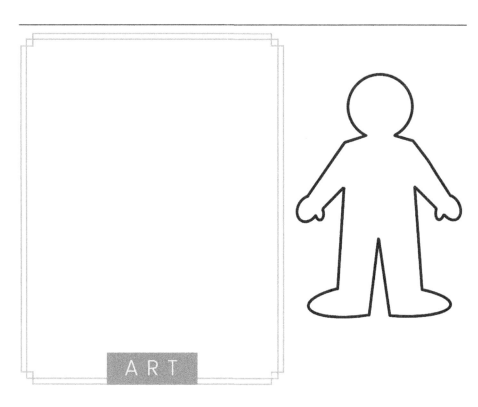

ART

date:_____

Today, I feel_____

about _____

_____

because_____

_____

I need_____

_____

I choose _____

_____

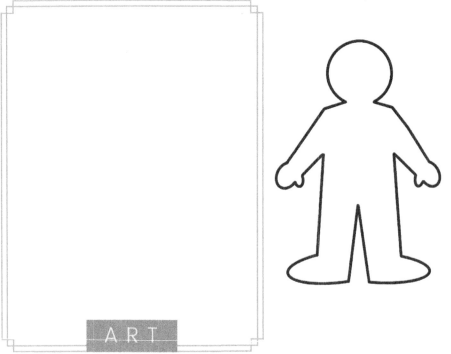

ART

date:_____

Today, I feel_____

about _____

_____

because_____

_____

I need_____

_____

I choose_____

_____

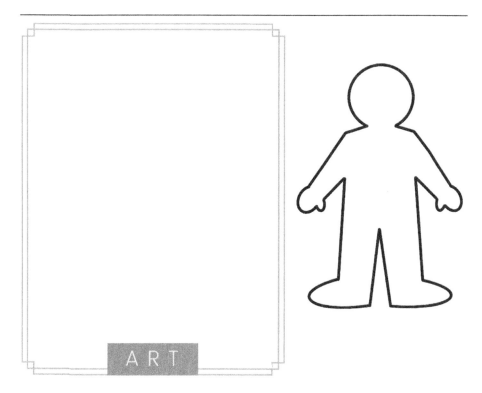

ART

date:_____

Today, I feel_____

about _____

_____

because_____

_____

I need_____

_____

I choose _____

_____

date:_____

Today, I feel_____

about _____

_____

because_____

_____

I need_____

_____

I choose _____

_____

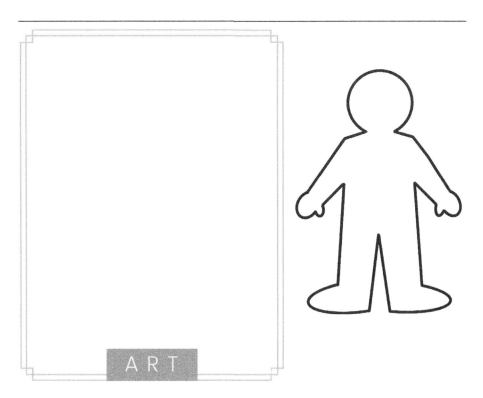

ART

date:_____

Today, I feel_____

about _____

_____

because_____

_____

I need_____

_____

I choose _____

_____

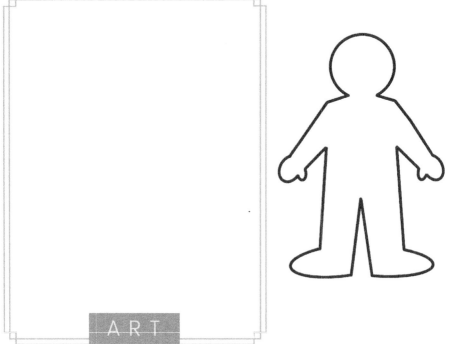

ART

date:_____

Today, I feel_____

about _____

_____

because_____

_____

I need_____

_____

I choose _____

_____

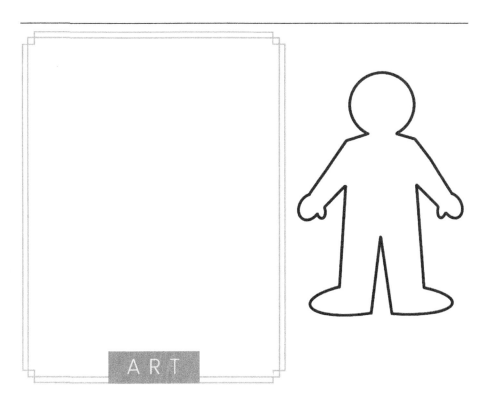

ART

date:_____

Today, I feel_____

about _____

_____

because_____

_____

I need_____

_____

I choose _____

_____

ART

date:_____

Today, I feel_____

about _____

_____

because_____

_____

I need_____

_____

I choose _____

_____

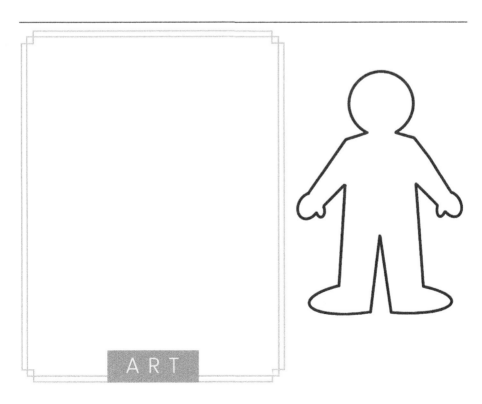

ART

date:_____

Today, I feel_____

about _____

_____

because_____

_____

I need_____

_____

I choose _____

_____

ART

date:_____

Today, I feel_____

about _____

_____

because_____

_____

I need_____

_____

I choose _____

_____

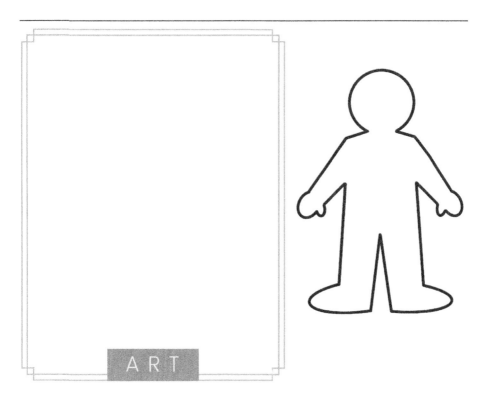

ART

date:_____

Today, I feel_____

about _____

_____

because_____

_____

I need_____

_____

I choose _____

_____

ART

date:_____

Today, I feel_____

about _____

_____

because_____

_____

I need_____

_____

I choose _____

_____

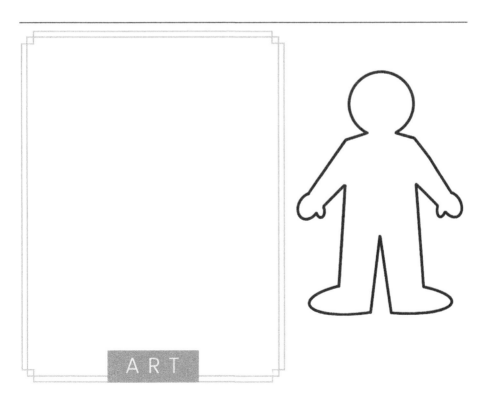

ART

date:_____

Today, I feel_____

about _____

_____

because_____

_____

I need_____

_____

I choose_____

_____

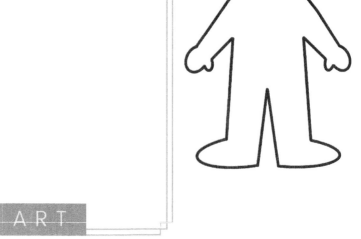

ART

date:_____

Today, I feel_____

about _____

_____

because_____

_____

I need_____

_____

I choose _____

_____

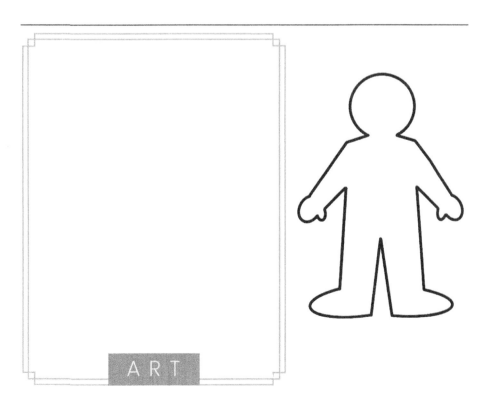

ART

date:_____

Today, I feel_____

about _____

_____

because_____

_____

I need_____

_____

I choose _____

_____

date:_____

Today, I feel_____

about _____

_____

because_____

_____

I need_____

_____

I choose _____

_____

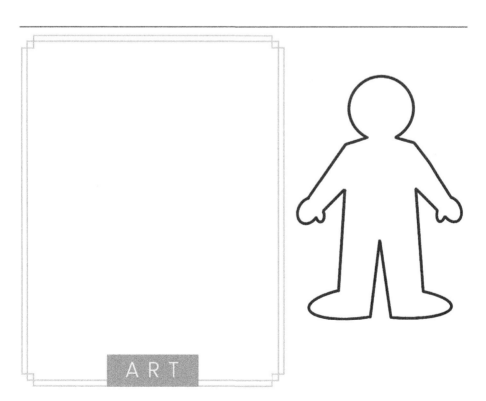

ART

date:_____

Today, I feel_____

about _____

_____

because_____

_____

I need_____

_____

I choose_____

_____

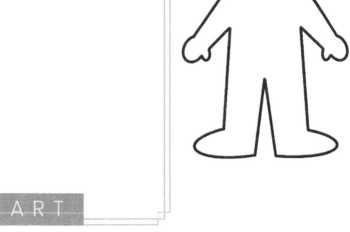

ART

date:_____

Today, I feel_____

about _____

_____

because_____

_____

I need_____

_____

I choose _____

_____

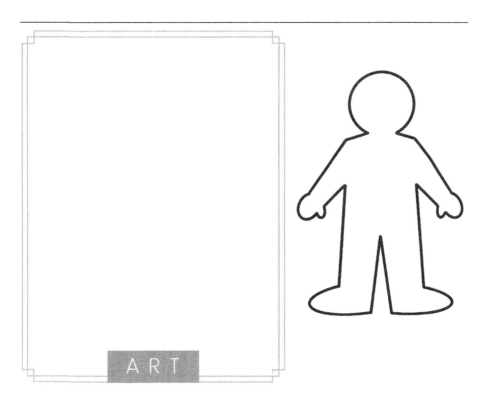

ART

date:_____

Today, I feel_____

about _____

_____

because_____

_____

I need_____

_____

I choose _____

_____

ART

Made in the USA
Coppell, TX
02 June 2023

17609381R00111